Read what others a
Doctor: Dr. Joe's RX for Managing Your Health

"Finally, here is a book of common sense and straight talk about the latest advances in health care for you, the patient. Learn self-care techniques now to prevent future problems. What does medicine of the future hold for you? How can you reverse the symptoms of illness? Dr. Joe did it. Find out how now."

> *Joan Palasota, Founder, B-Unlimited, Florida*

"Dr. Joe's personal story touched me deeply, and I learned what makes him a compassionate doctor, and a humanist in the field of medicine. He finally shares his personal discoveries with us, that we might become more active in the self-care movement and support patient education."

> *Tom Goode, ND, Author, Targeting an Optimum Lifestyle, how to stop killing yourself, Texas*

"Having to heal his own illness through pioneering approaches, Dr. Joe knows first hand what patients go through. His personal experience, wisdom, and wealth of information are finally compiled for you to read and use in *Dr. Joe's RX for Managing Your Health*."

> *Mark R. Rosales, President, CardioGrade. LLC, California*

The Uncommon Doctor: Dr. Joe's Rx for Managing Your Health

By
"Dr. Joe" Prendergast

The Uncommon Doctor:

Dr. Joe's Rx for Managing Your Health

By "Dr. Joe" Prendergast

© 2006 by Endocrine Therapeutics, Inc & Joseph Prendergast, MD

ISBN: 1-59975-022-8

ISBN13: 978-1-59975-022-4

Book Design & Publishing Assistance by
Nancy@WyMacPublishing.com

Index by Pueblo Indexing & Publishing Services
www.puebloindexing.com

Printed in Canada

Dedication

I dedicate this book to
Marlene,
Patrick
and
Peggy

Table of Contents

Acknowledgements

If you look at the history of diabetes, you see a cruel face. This book was written to compile the aspects of diabetes self-care into one source and to present you with a comprehensive overview and a successful program for managing your health and vitality. To achieve the personal goal of changing my life's arc involved patients, colleagues, staff, friends, and detractors. All made valuable contributions to this work, and I know they will continue to do so.

Many of these people have watched my transition from traditional endocrinology and metabolism care to my increasing role as an integrative medical practitioner. They have vetted each turn of philosophy knowing very well that they would likely be asked to personally participate in this change or at least defend it from the doubters. They have made valuable contributions to this book and I would like particularly to thank: Regis McKenna, author, friend and human being par excellence. He has worked with over 300 start-ups including Intel, Apple, Microsoft, and Genentech. Victor Dzau, MD, the person who startled me with the information that l-arginine could play a major role in reversing cardiovascular disease. He is now Chancellor for Health Affairs at Duke. John Cooke, MD, Professor of Medicine, Stanford School of Medicine, is a steadfast supporter of much of my clinical work and ever available to tutor me in my clinical research. Fred Whitehouse, MD, Director of the Diabetes Division at Henry Ford Hospital in Detroit enabled me to understand that I could make a difference in diabetes care and to trust me as I made my early decisions.

Special thanks to Penelope Mayes, RN, CDE, PHN, AS who is an incredible teacher and splendid communicator. She is director of major clinical projects, the success of which is due to her leadership and organizational skills.

Evelyn D. Castillo-Profeta, RN joined us by saying "I want to be best diabetic nurse in the US." Clearly, she is a finalist for that position.

Mark Rosales who helped me think about l-arginine as more than just medical treatment but a way of life for patients and their families. Joan Palasota opened many new pathways for me to enlarge my audience and encouraged me through each stage of this book.

All the gang at ForMor and especially Stan Goss and Michael Goss who convinced me I would do more good in the world if I would step outside my office. Lynn Camacho is the clinic manager who told me how I could really get things done and then did it all for me. And to all the rest of the members of the staff for all that you do for the patients.

I thank all the patients who questioned me hard and then trusted me with their future.

The invaluable experience of ghostwriter and psychologist, Caron Goode, Ed.D, provided the framework to write a book and then to get it done. I'd like to thank my editor, Sandra Mengine, proofreader and indexer, Gina Gerboth of Pueblo Indexing and Publishing Services, and book designer, Nancy Cleary of Wyatt-Mackenzie Publishing.

My wife Marlene gets special thanks for her support throughout all of the process and for her special editing skills.

Thanks to my daughter Peggy for her technical support and for the calming effect she has on me.

And, finally, thanks to my son Patrick for being so interested in the book project.

Foreword

I am honored to write the foreword for Dr. Joe Prendergast's new book, *Dr. Joe's RX for Managing Your Health*. I call Joe a revolutionary doctor and a pioneer because I have watched him lead the way in the holistic model of diabetic care throughout his career.

My relationship with Dr. Joe dates back to our early high school years where we both attended Cranbrook School for Boys in Bloomfield Hills, Michigan. Joe had been at Cranbrook a year before my arrival, and it was obvious at first glance, that Joe would be an outstanding leader, not only of our high school but throughout his life. I say "at first glance" because I observed Joe to be a hard working and dedicated individual, both in his academic achievements and extracurricular activities. You'll understand this outstanding accomplishment in academics when you read how Joe overcame a learning disability at a much later age than most children through focused study and hard work.

Joe put the same focus and effort into his athletic life by captaining both our football and baseball teams. He was appointed head prefect as the most outstanding individual in our graduating class, which ultimately included two Rhoades Scholars and a Heisman trophy winner in 1968.

Following his outstanding high school career, Joe

and I traveled to Williamstown, Massachusetts to attend a small liberal arts school, Williams College, where we roomed together for the next three years during our pre-medical training. The most poignant story which I remember had to do with the profound need for Joe, as a young man, to accept the loss of being forced to discontinue playing football as a freshman at Williams when he suffered the last of his many concussions. This would have taken a huge "hit" on his-self image in accepting this fact, for he had played it for so long and so well.

Football was now out of the question for Joe. But as life changes, so do the outcomes. Joe showed a formidable inner strength and found the resilience to change his focus. As Joe indicates in the book, at some expense to his Williams experience, he placed his energies in dealing with his family needs and his preparation for his life's work in medicine. So often, one event in life has meaning in other areas of our lives.

At Williams, Joe remained an excellent role model and I found him to be an exceptional roommate. Only my leaving Williams College following my third year to attend medical school served to split us as we went down slightly different pathways. I attended the University of Michigan and Joe attended Wayne State University Medical School. Since leaving Williams, I have maintained both a professional and a personal relationship with Joe over these past 45 years, watching his outstanding career grow year by year as he gained insight and developed leadership roles in the understanding, treatment, and education for diabetes mellitus. He recently received a prestigious award from the American Medical Association in March of 2005 for his outstanding research and his willingness to work with underprivileged Mexican-Americans, setting up an innovative telemedicine approach to specialty care in remote sites. He has served as the President of the Endocrine and Metabolic Medical Center and of the Pacific Medical Research Foundation. He has dedicated his entire career to furthering research and teaching within the field of diabetes. I am extremely proud to consider him a friend and a colleague. You will find within this book ways of effectively managing your own health.

Clifford W. Colwell Jr., MD

Medical Director and Clinical Professor of Orthopaedics and Rehabilitation at University of California at San Diego, Adjunct Professor at the Scripps Research Institute

La Jolla, CA, 92037

Introduction

The closer I got to the doors of the hospital, the more nervous I became. I had waited for this day for years and now all of my studying and practical training was about to pay off. For the first time, I was entering a hospital as a real physician. It was 1963, and I was starting my first rotation as an intern in the emergency room at William Beaumont Hospital in Royal Oak, Michigan. This was the real thing. I was a doctor! My blood ran high. I desperately wanted to serve my patients and make the best first impression possible to the staff. Most of all, I just didn't want to screw up.

I arrived at the hospital a few minutes early so I could introduce myself to everyone. I had a little speech that I gave to each doctor, nurse, and receptionist that went something like, "Hello. My name is Dr. Joe Prendergrast. I'm a new intern, fresh out of medical school. I don't know anything about this hospital, so I may ask you over and over how to get things done. If you see me going in the wrong direction, please let me know."

I had given my little spiel a few times and everything seemed to be going well. My confidence was growing. Suddenly, the doors of the emergency room burst open, and I saw a stretcher coming in from an ambulance. An enormous adrenaline rush shot through my body. Would I have to save this person's life? Before I could decide how to react, the ambulance driver announced that the woman on the stretcher was already dead.

That meant that my job would be to pronounce her dead. The very thought of doing it filled me with anxiety. As a medical student, I had seen plenty of dead bodies, and I had worked on cadavers, but the responsibility of ruling that a life has ended is serious business. Until now, it had always been someone else's job to make the monumental pronouncement. Very slowly, I began to carry out the procedures I had learned during my training. I checked her pulse and listened for a heartbeat. She was most certainly dead, but I didn't want to take any chances. I had visions of her sitting up in a casket four hours later saying, "Hey, I've got a terrible headache."

After making the pronouncement of death, it also fell to me to talk to her family about approving an autopsy. This was before CAT scans and diagnostic medicine, so her death had been a total surprise to the family. At that time, an autopsy was the only way to determine what had gone wrong; thankfully, they agreed to the procedure.

After speaking with them, my day melted into a more comfortable routine of treating coughs and sore throats. But the events of the morning still weighed heavily on my mind. Why had this relatively young woman of about 40 years of age died? Her family had mentioned that she was diabetic. I had never seen a diabetic before and wondered if the disease had played a role in her death.

Curiosity got the best of me, so later that afternoon I excused myself and went to see Dr. Jack Kevorkian perform the autopsy. That's right, the very same man who's now known internationally as "Dr. Death." However, at that time, he was simply known as a top-notch pathologist, and I was eager to learn from him.

I walked through the hospital until I found the place where the autopsy was underway. People are often surprised the first time they see the inside of an autopsy room. The space usually looks very similar to a typical operating suite, with good lighting and tables. The bodies are draped out of respect, just as they would be if they were alive and undergoing surgery.

When I entered the room that day, all I saw was Dr. Kevorkian bent over the body, performing what looked like abdominal surgery. I didn't say anything when I walked in. I simply stood there watching, not wanting to disturb his work. After a while, I became uncomfortable with the silence and thought about what I should say. How should I introduce myself to this serious doctor, so focused on the task at hand? Suddenly, he looked up from the body and said two words: "battery failure."

I was busy figuring out how to tell him that I was the new intern so the words "battery failure" seemed out of place and made absolutely no sense to me. I was too stunned to react. He must have noticed the confusion on my face because he explained, "Battery failure. Her pacemaker battery failed."

I grinned with relief. At least I now understood what he was talking about. With the silence broken, I peppered him with questions about the woman. In 1963, patients with pacemakers were not expected to live long enough to need a new battery. Her family had told me that she had a long history of diabetes. At this point, the disease was not well understood, and I certainly didn't know much about it. Dr. Kevorkian showed me evidence that she suffered from hardening of the arteries, which is a common sign of cardiovascular disease in people with diabetes.

Taking the opportunity to educate this young intern, Dr. Kevorkian asked me how many beta cells the woman had. Beta cells are insulin producers. She had what is now known as Type 1 diabetes, or insulin-dependent diabetes. Confidently, I told him that I knew the answer: I said, "None!" As a Type 1 diabetic, I figured she had no insulin production at all, therefore I thought she had no beta cells. I was crestfallen when he replied, "Wrong!"

Dr. Kevorkian took a sample of her pancreas. He said to come back the next day to see how many beta cells she really had in her body. As I traveled home that evening, the tension and anxiety I had felt during the day's events faded somewhat, but I still felt overwhelmed by everything I needed to learn if I was going to truly serve patients.

The next day, Dr. Kevorkian and I calculated that the woman had about 2,000 beta cells. That's a lot more than none, but still not nearly enough to maintain good health. The average person has one million beta cells. As we discussed her case, Dr. Kevorkian looked at me and said words I will never forget: "Someday you're going to find a way to make these cells grow." He said he didn't know how it was going to happen, but researchers would eventually figure out a way to increase the number of insulin-producing cells. He was right because that's what we do today.

Dr. Kevorkian showed me the woman's chart, and it appeared that she had received a lot of training on how to eat to treat her diabetes. At that time, doctors put diabetics on a very high-fat diet, thinking that the fat would delay the release of calories and insulin into the bloodstream. They believed that diabetes was only a problem with sugar, or glucose, and if you could slow the absorption of calories, you could control glucose levels. Dr. Kevorkian pointed out to me that he thought it was strange that physicians were using fat to treat a disease because it caused a host of other problems, including obesity, high cholesterol, and hardening of the arteries. Why treat one part of a disease in a way that just creates more disease? I was intrigued by what he had to say. It made me want to learn more about diabetes. There had to be a better way to help patients.

Later, in 1968, I saw the first glimmer of how diabetes treatment could be improved, and I agreed that it was completely wrong to increase the amount of fat in the diet. However, that first day with Dr. Kevorkian really started something for me. In fact, I realize that my first day as an intern shaped my entire medical career. Pronouncing that woman dead left me with unanswered questions. In the following years, even when diabetes was not the focus of my research, I never forgot her and continued to wonder what had led to her demise.

Over the next six months, I had frequent conversations with Dr. Kevorkian about how physicians should handle death as well as life. Whenever I had time, I would seek him out and he would stop what he was doing to speak to me. Today, he is still in jail in Michigan and I haven't talked to him in 35 years, but I'll never forget the intriguing questions he encouraged me to consider.

I had walked into the internship thinking, "I'm all done; I'm out of medical school and ready to roll!" In reality, I could not even imagine all I still needed to learn. On that first day of my internship, a whole new world opened to me. My conversations with Dr. Kevorkian and other doctors made me question everything I had learned. I realized that just because I had been taught something did not mean that it wouldn't be disproved as years went by. From that point on, I understood that "facts" must be accepted as only temporary knowledge and not absolute truths. Since then, I have seen this proven true many times, including the theory that diabetics should eat a high-fat diet. Keeping an open mind has been a guiding principal in my career, and I've become a better doctor and human being because of it.

I have never forgotten that there will always be new things to learn. Arrogance only stands in the way of true success. I once heard a story about how Walt Disney greeted the janitor on many mornings with a sincere inquiry on the state of Disneyland. After all, the janitor saw the park from a totally different perspective and surely noticed things that his boss would have missed. Like Mr. Disney, I have learned to embrace knowledge from every possible source. In all professions, including medicine, as soon as you think you know everything, you are in trouble.

My quest for knowledge has taken me to places in my professional and personal life that I could never have imagined that first day on the job. Over the last thirty years, I have conducted long hours of research in the field of diabetes and endocrinology. Dozens of articles about my work have appeared in numerous medical journals. I have also created the Pacific Medical Research Foundation through which I can further my vision of using the Internet to reach people without access to medical care. Most recently, in 2005, the American Medical Association honored me for working toward better understanding diabetes among disadvantaged populations in the United States.

I have accomplished many of my goals, despite having a learning disability that makes processing information more difficult for me. Learning to deal with my disability was not easy, and my struggles have made my accomplishments even more meaningful to me. While I take satisfaction in my successes, the real rewards have nothing to do with having money, a good reputation, or status within the medical community.

For me, the true excitement comes from learning more about the human body and facing new medical challenges. True gratification comes from living a life of service and leadership, and knowing that I have helped my patients and others struggling with diabetes. I live a fulfilling life by sticking to the same principles that I learned early in my life. They have served me so well; I would like to share them with you.

I am also writing this book to discuss the increasing problem of diabetes, which has reached epidemic proportions in our country. Each day, more than 2000 people in the United States are diagnosed with diabetes. This is a lifetime diagnosis with severe and potentially life-threatening complications. Unfortunately, for many reasons, some of these people will not receive the care they need. They will go through unnecessary pain and suffering because they will get substandard care, will not have access to the latest advances in diabetes management, won't know enough about their disease to engage in self-care, and will find themselves without a support network.

It doesn't have to be this way. People must know that so much of what we have learned or heard about diabetes in the past is no longer true. There are many new discoveries, like the use of l-arginine, that can dramatically improve, and even reverse, many of the complications suffered by diabetics. Most importantly, I want to share this message: If you have diabetes, you can take control, you can have a normal life, and you don't need to be limited in any way by your disease. For those of you who do not have diabetes, my message to you is the same. You can learn how to prevent yourself from ever contracting diabetes and other illnesses. You just need to know how.

John Joseph Prendergast, MD

October 4, 2005

CHAPTER 1

Lessons from My Childhood

Life on the farm felt like pure magic to a city kid like me, born on May 4, 1937 in Detroit, Michigan. My parents, Jack Prendergast, MD and Elizabeth Whitehead Prendergast, left the city and moved to a 160-acre farm in Dryden, thirty miles north of Detroit. I was about seven years old and wide-eyed when I saw the green and growing surroundings that hot summer. Our farm was what was then known as a "quarter of a square." This terminology dates back to a time when the entire Midwest was divided into squares, and farmers either got a whole square or a quarter square. Our farm was certainly not a huge farm, but everything about it seemed big to me.

I watched men lift enormous bales of hay and sacks of wheat. I thought that there was nothing the hired farm hands could not pick up or move, and I regarded them as heroic giants. After a morning of hard work, the men came in to wolf down what seemed like equally enormous lunches. Back then, lunch was called "dinner," and we called our evening meal "supper." I watched both the strength and appetites of the men with awe.

The area where we lived was still entirely an agrarian community, made up of farmers whose families had been working the land for many years. There were only two exceptions to this rule, our family and another family who had bought their farm a short time before we moved in. Our families stuck out. Our neighbors saw us as "city people," and it was true. As a boy from Detroit, I had a lot of new sites, sounds, smells, and ideas to get used to.

The closest thing to our farm was a gas station about two miles away. The nearest town, Dryden, was six miles away. I went to school there and all the area's social activities were held at the school. As a child, I had no way of traveling six miles to hang out with friends, so I mostly stayed at the farm and made my own entertainment like hunting and fishing. Rabbit hunting was especially exciting because it contained the social element of the men and dogs working together and the feeling of being part of a team. I also ran a trap line for muskrats, which earned me a little extra spending money. Of course, all of my pursuits were put on hold during harvest time. When the harvest came around, you harvested. There was not time for anything else.

Our farm could either feel like a place of solitude or isolation, depending on my mood and the weather. For the most part, I liked the peaceful quiet that came with living so closely tied to nature. Unlike my time in the city, I had almost total freedom to run and play. My imagination knew no boundaries. But sometimes I hated where we lived, especially as I got older. I remember many Friday nights when the bad roads forced me to miss a basketball game and I couldn't see my friends. When I think back to those frustrating evenings, I remember the snow and the mud, which forced us to cancel plenty of our already-rare social outings into town. During those times, I wished we had never left Detroit; but for the most part, I really enjoyed my childhood on the farm.

Living on the farm taught me a lot about the fragility of life. We didn't go to the grocery store for all of our meat and poultry. We knew the animals we consumed. On our farm, we raised turkeys and chickens. At one point, we had about 20,000 birds. One year, Newcastle's Disease came through our chicken farm and devastated us. We had to kill all of our chickens and then clean up the area, move the coops, and allow the ground to sit without any wildlife on it for several years. Even as a boy, it made me think about the rhythm of life and how much we don't know about the mysteries of nature. Viruses that we cannot predict or control can move in and dramatically change populations. I learned this tough lesson first by observing Newcastle's Disease, but the same can be said today about the bird flu or the emergence of SARS. No matter how much we know about medicine, nature and genetics will always exert control over our lives.

Living on the farm also taught me to rely on nature's rhythms to keep myself feeling healthy and balanced. As a boy, we got up with the sun and basically went to bed when it went down. Of course we had electric lights, but we relied on nature to set our clocks and determine when we worked. To this day, when I find that I'm overworked or stressed, I just go back to the natural rhythms of my childhood. A little exercise, adequate sleep, avoiding toxins found in food or alcohol, and avoiding bright lights in the night can suddenly put me right back on track. I can feel my body settle down quickly.

Life in our rural community helped me define many of the same principles I still value, including hard work, respect for nature, and leadership. From an early age, I felt a strong desire to contribute something to my school and my community. We were always taught that leadership and community support for the war was important. The first instance of this was in kindergarten when I was elected mayor of Pleasant Town. My teacher had come up with the idea of our classroom operating as a little village. Each student was assigned a different role in the community. I still remember the day I realized that somebody was going to be selected mayor and it might as well be me.

Of course, part of my desire to be mayor had to do with the developmental needs of a typical child. I wanted the recognition and validation that came with being chosen for what seemed to be a very important position in the classroom. However, I also wanted the chance to help my fellow students. I was sure that in my hands, the classroom could become a perfect little world.

One of the most exciting moments of my childhood came the day that our teacher read the ballot and I learned that I had been selected as mayor. I was sure that I would be able to influence the course of our school year and make Pleasant Town the best community ever. Looking back, it was a bit outlandish for a five-year-old to assume that he had the power to make real changes in school, but I was too naïve and determined to think any differently.

The Pleasant Town experience typified what was

going on in the country as a whole. We were in the middle of World War II, so everybody was talking about leadership. Adults told us that we had to be the best individuals we could possibly be because so much was going to be asked of us. This idea of individual responsibility struck a strong chord with me. When I decided I wanted to become the classroom's mayor, it was the first time that I realized that I might have the ability to be a leader. Once I started to serve in the position, I took the job very seriously. I remember standing in front of the class and trying to sound serious and authoritative as I made daily announcements. Some of the information was about the war. Of course, I wasn't reading the news or telling the kids, "Troops are invading Normandy." It was mostly about ways the children in our school could help the war effort by taking up collections to buy an airplane to give to the army.

I served my term as kindergartner mayor of Pleasant Town without any major excitement or incident, but the experience still influenced me greatly. From that point on, I felt driven to serve others by doing something, even if I couldn't always articulate what that "something" was. I worked hard to excel in the classroom and on the athletic field. Sure, I liked the feeling of being the best at something, but it was always about more than that for me. I truly wanted to give something of myself to those around me. As an adult, I still experience these exact same feelings every time I see a new patient in my office or find out about a new treatment for diabetes.

Looking back, I remember being a pretty good kid

living a pretty good childhood. However, like any kid, I had my share of problems and I got in more than a few fights. Saturday night was a big deal in Dryden. There was always some sort of social event and everyone would get dressed up, leave their farms for the evening, and head into town. I used to go with my parents and thought it was great fun, until I reached about the age of twelve. Even though we lived on a farm, my father was a doctor so some of the other kids labeled me as the "rich kid." For a few years, those bullies made me dread Saturday nights.

Whenever they would get the chance, usually when no adults were around, they would pick on me. It started with name-calling. Sometimes, it ended there, but often it turned into a fight. After the first physical attack, I realized that if I was truly going to be the person that I talked about, the leader, I had to change the way I faced these weekly confrontations. I knew that I couldn't win all of the fights because some of the kids were two years older and much bigger than I was. After stewing over the situation for a while, I came up with a plan. Even if I didn't win the fights, I would make sure that I never lost one. Somehow, I would hang in there until the kid fighting me would know that he had made a mistake. He too would take a terrible beating and realize he had picked on the wrong guy.

It didn't take long for me to put my plan into action. Sure enough, Saturday night arrived and the bullies approached me. One decided to prove that he was better than me, the little rich kid. For the first time, I stared down my nemesis with courage. I knew I couldn't beat him, but boy, was I going to make him pay for his decision. He started to punch me, and I just held tough. We fought it out to a draw. That boy never tried to fight me again.

Of course, that wasn't the end of it, not by a long shot. I faced down many more bullies of different ages and sizes, but the end result was always the same: I never lost! It took about ten fights ending in a draw for the bullying to stop, but eventually it was over. In each case, it was my attacker, not me, who walked away.

I had learned an important principal in my life that I still employ as an adult. I will not be beaten when something is important to me. Fortunately, I don't have to apply it so literally today. I don't find myself in fistfights anymore. Yet, no matter what the situation is, I hang tough.

I also learned that hanging tough and being the aggressor are two very different things. During this time, there was a boy who was about my age who liked to pick on me. One day, I decided that I had listened to enough and I hit him. For the first time, I was the one who started the physical fight. I lashed out partly because I was enraged by his words, but also because I was emboldened by my new experiences in fighting. I made a big mistake. Apparently, this kid had the same determination not to be beaten. I did my best to knock him down and he refused to give in. The fight ended in a draw, just like the other ones.

We were both about the same size so neither one of us really hurt the other. However, this time I was the big loser. I had attacked someone. That night, I went home feeling embarrassed and ashamed. After all, I had made the wrong choice and had acted as badly as all of the other guys who had bullied me. That was the last time I ever tried to use physical aggression to solve a problem.

My Father's Influence

My experience dealing with bullies helped shape me into the adult I am today. I also went to some good schools and had some excellent teachers. But no one shaped my outlook on life like my father. He is the main reason that I developed an intense desire to succeed through helping others.

Like every family, we had our share of problems and little secrets. We moved out of Detroit and to the farm largely because my mother was an alcoholic. My parents thought she would fare better in the rural environment, but it didn't really work. She continued to drink heavily throughout my childhood. Because of her struggles, I relied even more on my father to guide me. He certainly never let me down. To this day, I can't think about him without feeling a bit choked up.

What a guy my dad was! During much of my childhood, my father, Dr. Jack Prendergast, was the medical director of Chrysler Corporation. It was a good, respectable job. The sheer will it took my father to get to the point where he accepted that job still seems like a miracle to me. Dad came from an Irish Catholic family. As an adult, he didn't attend church services often, but the principles of the church, including honesty and compassion, stayed with him throughout his life.

He was born in 1901 and grew up in West Virginia.

When he was a teenager, his father pulled some strings for him and got him a job as a gandy dancer for the Baltimore and Ohio Railroad. Gandy dancers laid track and helped maintain the lines. It was considered a good job for a boy his age, but my father was determined to achieve more. When he was about 18, he told his family that he was leaving to go to medical school. While that may sound like something parents would love to hear from an ambitious son, my grandparents thought such dreams were out of the realm of possibility. They became so angered that he could even consider leaving a steady job that they threw him out of the house and refused to speak to him.

Undeterred, my father headed to Buffalo, New York and got into college. He supported himself by playing professional basketball. It was a different era and playing professional sports did not have near the cache it has today. Still, he made enough money that he was able to put himself through an undergraduate program and ultimately through medical school. Once he graduated, he decided he wanted to be an OBGYN at Detroit Receiving Hospital. He went to apply for the job, but the head of the department immediately turned my father down, telling him he wasn't interested.

My dad then did something that speaks volumes about the kind of guy he was. He looked at the head of the department and said, "Fine. Okay. Then I'd like the job as an orderly. I'll just clean up after you guys. I really want this position because it will allow me to learn from what you are doing." Later, my father told me that the doctor gave him a weird look and said, "Okay smart guy, be the orderly."

His career as an orderly lasted about two weeks. The same man, who had turned him down at first, gave him a position as a resident in the OBGYN Program. He ultimately became the Chief Resident of OBGYN. When I was growing up, I often thought of my dad's determination, and it motivated me to push harder for success in my own life.

The way he got his first job as a doctor is a great story that I love retelling, but it doesn't surprise anyone who knew my dad. He always focused on pursuing his interests in a way that would help other people. No job was too small for him if it served a common good. I became a doctor largely because of my father's influence, but he never really cared what career path I took. He only cared how I conducted my life. He would say to me, "If you are a carpenter, do the best job possible. If you're a banker, be the best banker you can be. That's what matters."

Later in his career, he was offered the position as medical director at Chrysler. At the time, it was a very progressive idea in the auto industry. No company had ever hired a medical director before. He worked very hard and shaped the position to fit his vision. Slowly, all of the companies began to hire medical directors, but my father was the first in the industry.

There is a part of my father's career that I still don't know much about. During World War II, he was part of the Manhattan Project, a World War II program that focused on developing the United States' first atomic bomb. Even until his death, he never told me much about that period in his life, but he indicated that he was trying to come up with ways to protect the workers responsible for making the bombs.

When I was 19, my father died, leaving a void in my life that could not be filled. I knew he was in poor health, but his death was still a tremendous shock. Looking back, he had some habits, including smoking, that must have negatively impacted his health. He also probably had a genetic predisposition to develop heart disease. I know this, because I was diagnosed with the same condition. However, I have benefited from medical knowledge that my father never lived to know. Later, in this book, I'll tell you how I was able to reverse the heart disease that killed my father.

My dad's physical decline started with a series of strokes. The first occurred when he was 42 years old when I was a freshman at boarding school. After that stroke, he never really worked again. Seeing my father ill was tough for me to come to terms with as a teen. I had only known him as a dynamic force within our family and his profession. His work ethic and service to others resonated with me and made me want to be like him. He was so important to many lives, not just mine.

Over the years, people have come up to me and said the most extraordinary things about his influence on them. I've been told, "Everything I achieved in life I owe to your father," "He gave me a job when no one else would," and "He believed in me." To this day, I am more proud of him then I will ever be able to adequately express. I am also so grateful to him for giving me a set of core values that has served me throughout my life.

CHAPTER 2

Cranbrook School

Next to my father, nothing influenced me as a young man as much as my time spent in boarding school. When I was 14, my parents sent me to Cranbrook School in Bloomfield Hills, Michigan, about 40 miles from our farm. My parents wanted to insure a good education for me, and if I didn't go to Cranbrook, I would have gone to our local high school. At that time, there was only one person in the history of our local high school that had gone to college, as the school was obviously not geared toward an academic track of any kind. Because I wanted to go to college, my parents and I agreed that Cranbrook seemed like the best solution.

I wanted to go, but boy, was I scared. Just getting accepted into the program was intimidating as one had to go through a series of interviews and take examinations. I took part in a group interview with other kids who sat in the library and waited for the teachers to question us. Looking around the room, the other guys seemed like seven-foot-tall geniuses. Some of the boys were saying, "Well, I'm going to first take my collegiate work at Harvard. From there I'll complete a Master's degree at Princeton, and then I'll go to med school at Columbia." I was floored. I thought, "Good God, these guys have planned out their whole lives, and I don't even know what I'm doing tomorrow!"

The summer before I was to start at Cranbrook, I took the required tests and I did horribly. The administrators told me that I would have to repeat the eighth grade. I was crushed. I didn't want to have to go back and spend another year in my old school. My parents and I asked if there was an alternative. They said, "Well you could tutor with one of the math teachers and perhaps read some other material that would bring you up to the level of the other students." I immediately agreed to try that.

Looking back, it is not surprising that I didn't meet Cranbrook's admittance standards. Not only did I not do well on tests, the local school had left me woefully unprepared for a real academic environment. For instance, I was supposed to be competent in algebra, yet I had never ever heard the word "algebra." I worked hard over the summer and finally the big day came for me to leave home and head to Cranbrook. I walked into the school's beautiful courtyard, feeling scared stiff. My dad sort of said, "Here you are. See you later." Actually, I'm sure he said at least a little more than that, but at the time, I felt completely abandoned. I stood there, nervously clutching a suitcase holding just a handful of clothing. As I stared at the other students and the lovely buildings carefully modeled after the Cranbrook School in England, I wondered what kind of administrative error had led to my acceptance. Did I really belong in this place? It was intimidating.

However, as my first day progressed, the teachers I met were extremely friendly and supportive, and I didn't see any of the guys I had interviewed with. In fact, once I started to talk to other students, they all seemed like average teenagers, just like me.

Cranbrook is a physically beautiful place and a serene environment for a young person. I soon adjusted to my new life and felt at home. At home, I was used to being bullied and teased. By the end of my four years at Cranbrook, I had become president of the class and co-captain of the football team. Talk about a boost in self-esteem!

Athletic ability had always come naturally to me, but I had never played on an organized sports team until I got to Cranbrook. I joined the freshman football team as a left halfback. Our team did really well and won most of our games. It put a little swagger in my walk.

Later that school year, I also joined the varsity baseball team. That was the team to be on! Our families would give us cars for four weeks or so and we would drive from Michigan to North Carolina for spring training. That's right, spring training for high school students! We would stay in freshman visiting-team dorms and play freshman teams. All of the coaches we ran into told us what a good team we were. It was such an exciting time. We really thought we were hot shots. My sense of self-worth soared during my first season on the baseball team.

I had also planned to play basketball, but I had suffered a minor injury in football, so I couldn't try out for the team. This was a big letdown because my friends played all three sports. A new season meant a new sport. The quarterback on our football team, Peter Dawkins, had also gotten hurt. We were steamed! I said to a coach, "Well, we can't play, but we don't want to sit around in study hall. What can we do?" He suggested that we just run. It sounded weird, but we tried it and loved it.

Peter later went on to win the Heisman Trophy at West Point, and became nationally known for his military career, but we joke that our biggest accomplishment is that we invented jogging. After all, no one ran for fun at that time. We didn't copyright jogging, but in our hearts, we know it is our discovery. We like to kid around and tell people that we have made a huge contribution to the world by giving humankind the gift of jogging. Of course, everyone looks at us like we are crazy, but that's okay.

While I excelled at sports, scholastics did not come nearly as easily for me. In fact, I only earned a D average on my first report card. The headmaster, Harry Hoey, wrote to my parents, "Not much of a scholar, but I guess a fair athlete." My Latin teacher told me, "You shouldn't be getting grades like this!" I was devastated. To me, my report card was solid proof that I was stupid. There could be no other explanation. After all, I wasn't being lazy and I really felt like I was trying to do well. I made a resolution to work even harder. I spent long hours studying, trying to improve my grades. The faculty at Cranbrook believed in me and supported me in more ways than I can mention. Instead of lectures, I received encouragement. In the second report card sent to my parents, Mr. Hoey commented that I was improving and was even developing some leadership potential.

Still, despite my best efforts, I could never pull

straight A's. I made it into the top third of the class, but I was always in the bottom half of the top third. Sometimes, it felt very discouraging to know that I was trying; yet I couldn't achieve the excellent grades that seemed to come so easily to other boys. I decided that maybe I wasn't that smart, but I would make up for it with determination. By the end of the year, I did manage to get an A in Latin, but it was only through rote memorization.

All of the students at the school had their own rooms. Each night, after dinner in the dining hall, we had to come back and study for several hours. Some kids hated the regimented study program, but I liked it. It was the only thing that helped me improve my grades. Still, even when my test scores got better, I was convinced that I just wasn't as smart as the other guys at Cranbrook.

The next few years at Cranbrook flew by. I had to work hard to get decent grades, but it paid off. Improving my grade point average gave me the confidence to keep going. As a high school student, I really came to understand that if I worked hard, I could excel at academics. I grew to love Cranbrook and thrived on the consistent encouragement and support I received there.

At the end of my junior year, the schoolmasters picked students to serve as "prefects." Each house had a prefect who led his group in various activities. The masters selected the prefects based on their leadership potential. Then, out of all of the prefects, they named a head prefect. They gave that job to me. When I was told that I was chosen, I was astounded and more than proud. Becoming head prefect was the highlight of my young life.

I had gone from the kid who almost had to repeat the eighth grade to the head of the student body. Later at graduation, I received the school's Good Citizenship Award. Not only had I done well in academics and sports, I had been a good citizen of the school. This recognition made me feel like there was nothing I could not accomplish.

During this time, I received a lot of encouragement from my father. He had a stroke in the spring of my freshman year, so he wasn't completely mobile. Still, he made it to as many of my games as he could. When I was getting bad grades, there were times when I wanted to give up. I would tell him that maybe Cranbrook was just too much for me. Maybe I should become a farmer. He would look me straight in the eye and say, "No, you've got plenty of ability. You'll be there. You'll catch up. Don't worry about it." My friends and experiences at Cranbrook influenced me and shaped me, but my father's belief in me kept me going. His unwavering confidence sustained me through some difficult times.

My Surprise Diagnosis

I worked hard and learned to live with not getting perfect grades. Still, I often wondered why, despite all of my achievements and strengths, processing information could be so difficult. It wasn't until I had completed all of my medical training that I learned the secret behind my troubles in school. I have a learning disability. It is associated with an inherited disorder called "galactosemia trait" that prevents me from learning in the same way that most people do.

Galactosemia trait is a metabolic disorder, which is caused by an enzyme deficiency. This deficiency impairs the body's ability to use the simple sugar galactose. It causes an accumulation, and therefore high levels, of galactose 1-phosphate. This is not the same as the sugar problems that occur with diabetes. However, both disorders share some of the same complications. In both cases, high levels of sugar can damage the liver, central nervous system, and various other bodily systems. Galactosemia trait is especially problematic for women because it can damage the ovaries and cause early menopause. In addition to all of these complications, it can also cause specific learning disabilities.

It never even occurred to me that I could have galactosemia trait, much less a learning disability! I never suspected that I had a problem until my daughter was diagnosed with galactosemia trait. She had been identified very early as a mentally gifted minor. In spite of the fact that she was highly intelligent, she did not do well in the advanced placement courses. They tested her to see what was wrong. After years of underperformance and the inability of experts to solve the problem, medical experts determined that she had galactosemia trait, which greatly affected her ability to concentrate, read, and test on abstract concepts. With this, a light bulb went on in my head. I thought, "That is my problem too!" It all added up.

My daughter was only the 292nd person to ever be diagnosed with galactosemia trait. When I was tested, I became the 293rd. Although it is a rare condition, experts believe most of the people who suffer from it are never diagnosed. Therefore, I now test all of my patients for galactosemia trait.

My daughter and I both have a hard time taking tests, especially ones involving math. Part of my problem with processing information is physical. I have a visual impairment where I don't see well in fluorescent light. It takes me longer to understand what is in front of me.

However, my daughter and I are very good at seeing things spatially. When we are confronted with new scenario, we are able to grasp the big picture quickly and assess what is wrong or right about the situation. Therefore, on any given subject, we might not test well, but if we were graded based on a conversation about the subject, we would score well above average. For instance, when I got to medical school, I had a really hard time with all of the bookwork. However, once we got into the clinical years, I shot to the top of the class. Even now, I can walk into an office with only a handful of data on a patient and within seconds of meeting them, figure out exactly the treatment they need. Ironically, the disability that almost made me repeat the eighth grade has made me a better doctor.

When I was at Cranbrook, galactosemia trait also made me a better football player. Within a millisecond, I could accurately assess where everybody was on the field and which direction they were moving. People would ask me, "How is it that you seem to know where to run almost before you've seen all of the players?" I would tell them I didn't know, which was true at the time. It is only now that I see the way I learn has drawbacks, but it also has benefits.

Not knowing that I had a learning disability was tough because I always assumed I was dumb. Newborns weren't screened for galactosemia trait until 1963. So many people are still living their lives not even knowing they have it. Although I firmly believe in proper diagnosis of learning disabilities, in some ways I also think I benefited from not knowing about it. Since I never knew that I had a valid reason for my poor scores, it never occurred to me to make excuses for my grades. I simply made myself work harder than my classmates.

Returning to Cranbrook

Trying to compete with my classmates was never easy, and it still isn't! I had the good fortune to go to school with some exceptional people. Our graduating class included two eventual Rhodes scholars and others who achieved at very high levels. Recently, we all got together for our 50th class reunion. I was amazed at the varied and fascinating careers in our group. One of the men became a real superstar in the legal profession. Another helped negotiate for the hostages during the Carter administration. Dr. Colwell, who wrote the foreword for this book, is another. Many of my former schoolmates have shown remarkable leadership qualities, which I believe they developed at Cranbrook.

Several years ago, I had a chance to return to Cranbrook to give the commencement address. Much has changed at the school, especially with the rapid onset of new technology. Cranbrook is now a co-ed school. It was fun to see the differences and the many things that are still the same. Cranbrook is still doing an excellent job of providing students with strong academic and moral foundations that will serve them throughout their lives. Standing in front of the graduating class, I knew that I could not even imagine the many paths their lives would take. However, I wanted to let them know that they could succeed through leadership, even when facing tremendous obstacles. I told them:

When I left Cranbrook the essence of leader-ship was to be of good moral character, work hard, know your goals, and if you stood up straight you would prevail. This probably never was enough then, but it surely is not enough now.

Today, leadership first depends on your ability to make rapid decisions, often with inadequate information. It seems everything should have been completed yesterday. Couple this with the full alert for discordance in the midst of this accelerated compression of the decision time space. This is critical. The need for this kind of decision analysis has always been exciting in the medical field. Now it's everywhere.

Remember that as a leader you have a moral duty to be a revolutionary. Keep your intellectual footing secure, based in evidence, not assumptions. As information sharing nears warp speed it is much easier to test basic assumptions. Your education has given you a solid base of understanding of leadership inter-action in society, and now you are poised to seek your niche in the world.

While you're at it, aim high. If you fail, as I have, fail with something really good, something ahead of its time. Be a pioneer. Get out in front. The middle ground is an exposed, dangerous, ungrateful position.

Throughout your time you will have

to conform to the rules, but beware the tyranny of conformity. It is a pivotal concept that you must carry with you. Keep a little doubt that work done before you was done correctly. I remember when the placebo effect was assumed to be correct. Recent data indicates that this effect has never been proven. I have been involved in over 200 medical research projects in which the placebo figured in the basic study design. What are we to do now that it's gone?

As you start new projects, there is really no way to reassure yourself that what you are doing is not self-delusional. But remember too that a smaller mind than yours with a stingier conscience would not have even started.

Doing a new thing is a lot like bull fighting. You are either in the emergency room or on center stage. But for all the good you will try to do, you can still look forward to the bite of a vengeful, talentless man on your way to develop something potent, serious, successful.

So believe in yourself as you grow your skills and your life. The leadership you bring to all that you do will add authenticity to your whole career. Your innovation nurtures the luster of all your good ideas, constantly polishing up your image to its true gleam, the way it's supposed to be.

I delivered this message of insightful leadership to Cranbrook School graduates about their lives. However, the theme also pertains to your role in managing your health and quality of life. Step forth in this information age to gain new knowledge about what programs, research, or strategies can improve your physical well-being. I'll share more about breakthroughs in the wellness field as we move along.

The important point is that you should take charge of your health through every stage of your life. You will not have the time to have an understanding of acute illness or injury but as you go along in life you must develop healthy life patterns. If you have developed a chronic disease such as diabetes you should develop healthy life patterns tailored to your problem. Disease has been demystified and the treatments are not magical. Ask any search engine for the basics and ask that you receive updates on published material. You must take the lead in education. How else will you know what questions to ask? I got bad grades as I started in life but worked hard to learn. If you have developed a chronic disorder you must learn too. It's your time.

CHAPTER 3

Losing My Support System

Little did I know how much my world was about to change when I graduated from Cranbrook. I felt like I was ready to take on the world, optimistic about my future and excited to be going to college. While attending Williams College in Williamstown, Massachusetts, my father died. Shortly after I finished at Williams, my mother died. What I thought would be a time of great excitement turned into one of the most difficult and emotionally draining periods of my life.

I hadn't been at school for very long when I got word that my father had passed away. Suddenly, my main support system was gone. Even though Dad had been physically disabled for a number of years before his death, mentally he had continued to be as sharp as ever. I was ready to launch into another four years of school, but this time I would have to do it without my mentor and role model. Over the next four years, there would be so many times that I wished I could talk to my dad.

Before my father's death, my family moved to Florida for the better climate. I stayed behind to go to college. My mother had never really stopped drinking, and my father's death prompted her to drink even more. She suffered from a lot of health problems, including pancreatitis, which eventually killed her. Losing her was another blow. Although she had become ineffective as a parent, I still loved her and was devastated by her death. I was legally an adult, but I felt like an orphan.

It was even worse for my siblings. My brother was still in high school when our parents died. My sister had just graduated from college and was working in Washington D.C. She made the brave decision to give up her job and the life she was creating and move to Florida to care for my brother. I felt a tremendous amount of guilt and confusion. Here she was, giving up her new career, and I was going on with my education as planned. I wondered if I should also go to Florida to be with them, but that would mean dropping out of school. We made the decision as a family that I would continue my education, but it was not easy for any of us. I still get a little emotional when I think about it.

Even before my father died, I had not been able to visit my family that much in Florida. In those days, you couldn't just jump on a plane and fly down for the weekend. Visiting meant driving four to six hours on narrow, winding roads to Boston or New York, then flying to Florida and trying to find transportation to the house. Not only was the trip a struggle, I couldn't afford to travel. My father had left trusts for our educations, but I had very little money for anything else.

So I stayed at school, but my mind was constantly with my family. I worried about them and dwelled on my feelings of guilt for not doing more for my younger brother. There was the lingering feeling that I was somehow sucking away the family's money. Even though I had a scholarship, my education was expensive. However, the bank assured me many times that I was not compromising my siblings' inheritance. Dad had several years to prepare for his death and he had done a good job of setting up trusts for our education. Still, even with my brother and sister telling me to continue with college and medical school, I never felt completely at peace with our arrangement. All three of us felt responsible for each other, and I lived with the feeling that I wasn't fulfilling my family obligations.

I went through my four years at Williams College often feeling isolated and depressed. Williams College had seemed like the right place for me. After all, it was a good school and many of my idols from Cranbrook had gone there. I had also deliberately picked the school because of its rural setting. Since I had grown up on a farm, I figured the solitude would be comforting. At that point, I hadn't had many city experiences and I didn't want any distractions. Also, like Cranbrook at that time, it was a school for males only. I figured that going to a co-ed college would make it harder to focus. Considering my trouble getting decent grades, having a big social life seemed like a mistake.

I got what I wanted, a solid education with minimal distractions, but I also gave up a lot. One bright spot at Williams was getting to know the school's chaplain. Sloan Coffin was the first person I ever met who truly seemed to live a life of Christ. He loved all people, no matter their race or background. Even though I didn't consider myself particularly religious, the idea of leading a life devoted to God had fascinated me since elementary school. I was very interested in religion.

In fact, as a child, I thought that I would eventually become a Jesuit priest. The idea of the priesthood appealed to me because I liked the concept of living according to strongly held principles. By the time I was fourteen, I had changed my mind and no longer wanted to enter the priesthood. However, I still was involved in church. At Cranbrook, I read scriptures during Sunday services. Although I didn't feel overly connected to the church, I loved trying to communicate the messages of the Bible in a way that would be meaningful to my fellow classmates. It felt great to be of service.

Reverend Coffin often used to come to our fraternity house for dinner. One time, while he was eating with us, someone took a shotgun and fired a bullet through his living room window. Apparently not everyone appreciated his love for all people, including African-Americans. I was incensed by the hatred and stupidity behind such an act. To my amazement, he seemed to take the attack in stride.

I said to him, "I just can't be a real Christian like you. I just don't have it in me. I can't get over the fact that if someone hits me in the face I should just say 'nice swing' and turn the other cheek." He looked at me with compassion, but didn't respond. Trying to get my point across, I elaborated by saying, "I really admire what you've done and I've learned a huge amount from you, but I'm going to continue on my path of being a physician. In that capacity, I'll carve out my own life. But, it won't be the life of Christ that you're living."

I wondered if I had said too much. Had I insulted him and his calling? But, he replied, "That's wonderful. You're doing it just right." Reverend Coffin's encouragement made me even surer that I wanted to pursue a career in medicine. While I admired members of the clergy, he helped me see that I could apply the same principals of dedication and service to a career in medicine.

In retrospect, I'm sure that the fact that my father was a physician was also one of the reasons I chose to become a doctor. However, when I entered Williams, I didn't really know what I wanted to be. It's not like I was walking around Cranbrook telling people I was going to work in medicine. In fact, I liked the idea of becoming a forest ranger. I imagined myself spending my days hiking through the woods, looking at plants and animals. It seemed like a peaceful way to live. But there comes a time in every college student's life when you have to declare a major. The school asked me what mine would be and I blurted out, "Well, I'd like to be a doctor." That was it! I had just chosen a career. It was such a sudden decision. I am still not sure what made me say those words, but in retrospect, it all fit.

Medical School

After Williams College, I went to medical school at Wayne State University in Detroit. It was a really good experience. My mother died the first few months of medical school. With that final loss, I began to adjust to not having parental support.

My still-undiagnosed learning disability made the first two years of course work extremely difficult. The first year was especially hard because we learned almost nothing but anatomy. However, I studied relentlessly and managed to get satisfactory grades. During the second year, we were able to take paying jobs in the hospital. We were responsible for taking histories and giving physicals to people who had been admitted into the hospital. Afterwards, the medical students would meet with the practicing doctors in the cafeteria. We would eat and discuss our patients. The doctors would tell us how their day had gone. It was so exciting! Although my daytime classes continued to be tough, I learned very quickly on the job.

The last two years of medical school were even more inspiring. We got away from the textbooks and increased our practical training. I didn't have to study at all. Everything just seemed to come to me. I was thrilled to be absorbing knowledge so quickly. Instead of putting facts into my brain that I would have to retrieve during an exam, I could now see how all of the pieces of information that I had been learning fit together like a big puzzle. Everyday, a light bulb went on in my head. Many times during my hospital work I jubilantly exclaimed, "Oh, this is why we learned this! Yes, I understand now!" Finally, I felt like I was doing exactly what I was meant to do. Medicine began to truly feel like my calling.

Every third night, the hospital allowed six medical students to spend all night working in the emergency room. They were coveted jobs and I was lucky enough to get one. Most nights, there wasn't much going on. It was a tiny, quiet hospital. However, sometimes we got to help patients who had suffered massive injuries from strokes, car accidents, or gunshot wounds. The other students and I could ask the attending physicians questions and get feedback on our performance. It was wonderful because the six of us got so much more experience than the other students, allowing us to learn at a much faster rate. The long hours made us tired but better prepared for our upcoming internships.

To be honest, the nights spent in the emergency room made me feel a little cocky. After so many years of struggling to understand schoolwork, I loved being able to perform so well. In some ways, it felt like I was back running on the football field at Cranbrook. In the fast-paced ER, I immediately grasped the important elements of the situation and knew how to respond. I got excellent feedback from my supervisors and peers, so I knew I was doing a good job.

After medical school, I completed my internship at

William Beaumont Hospital. Dealing with the death of a diabetic patient on my first day sparked my interest in the disease. But it was not my main focus and I didn't think I would specialize in the treatment of diabetes. After William Beaumont Hospital, I went to Henry Ford Hospital in downtown Detroit, where I finished a fellowship in endocrinology and metabolism.

At Henry Ford, I became Chief Resident and spent two years supervising the training of 200 younger physicians. I organized regular classes. However, I also continued to find other ways to make our learning more meaningful. For instance, I hosted luncheons where we bet our paychecks on how we could manage a certain patient most effectively. Bouncing ideas off of each other turned out to be satisfying for both new and more experienced residents alike. Still, even in my leadership role, I always worried that I hadn't learned enough to give patients the care they needed. The realization that the human body is still largely a mystery kept me from getting arrogant or too sure of myself.

CHAPTER 4

*The Detroit Riots:
Changing My Perspective*

In 1967, I had been working as a doctor for a few years when the riots occurred in Detroit. The mayhem in Detroit was one of the several race riots to break out in America that summer. The riot started at an after-hours club in a mostly black neighborhood in the Northwest side of the city. The police showed up and found 82 people celebrating at a party for a couple of Vietnam veterans who had just come home. The officers started making arrests and crowds began to protest immediately. Looking back, it isn't surprising that a race riot happened in Detroit. After several high-profile cases of police brutality against black residents, there was terrible tension between cops and those they were supposed to be protecting. Add to the mix the many forms of political, social, and economic injustice against blacks at that time, and an outbreak seemed inevitable.

As the police waited for backup to help take away those they had arrested, two people in the crowd broke into a clothing store. They claimed they had no place else to go. Their actions sparked a wave of looting and fires throughout the city that lasted for five days. When the violent rampage was over, 43 people were dead and nearly 1,200 were injured. Police reported making 7,000 arrests. The National Guard and 82nd Airborne had to help get the riot under control.

With so many incoming injured, Henry Ford Hospital experienced mayhem. Anyone with any sense working at the hospital went home. I stayed. For those five days, I was basically in charge of the hospital. Not only was the staff inundated with emergency patients, we also were under constant assault from the outside. Bullets were bouncing off of the building. Everyone on the staff experienced true terror.

During those five days, we almost never got a break. In the day, we would try to get a little sleep because each night was chaotic. The gunshot victims seemed to never stop coming. On several occasions we had children die in the emergency room. Most of them had been standing around and were hit by stray bullets. To see them make it to the hospital and then have their hearts stop was terrible, but everything was happening so quickly, we could barely process the pain. Before a death could sink in, more stretchers would be coming through the doors.

Several nurses would stay by the doors and screen everyone who showed up. If it was serious they would scream, "We need a doctor, right now!" Most of the doctors were too busy suturing patients, so as the supervisor I would drop what I was doing and run to answer their call for help.

On the fifth day, I was at the door with two nurses, and we had just screened a few young black men with gunshot wounds. Like many of the patients, they were simply innocent bystanders, in the wrong place at the wrong time. As they were wheeled into the emergency room, we all fell apart. We just didn't have it in us anymore. We were drained. At that point, I didn't know how the staff could see even one more patient. None of us had the strength to do it again. We helplessly looked at each other, feeling a terrible mix of fear and exhaustion. How could we help anyone else? It was one of the worst moments of my life.

Miraculously, no more patients came. The riots were over. Unbeknownst to us, we had collapsed only after reaching the finish line. But we were too numb from sadness and fatigue to feel any relief or to congratulate ourselves on not giving up.

Working with those fine nurses during the riots gave me a new perspective on the field of nursing. I had always appreciated nurses' hard work and enormous contribution to patient care. In many ways I was a young doctor too consumed with my own responsibilities to appreciate the amount of teamwork it takes to effectively run a hospital. Our work during the riots taught me a valuable lesson about the skills and compassion required to be a top-notch nurse. Since then, I have had the honor of working with many fantastic nurses. My deep respect for their profession has only increased over the years.

On August 1, 1967, Mayor Jerome Cavanagh, Michigan Governor George Romney, and the president of the JL Hudson department store chain announced the formation of the New Detroit Committee. The goal was to bring together community leaders from around the city to ease the social problems that had contributed to the riots. The members of the committee included the heads of General Motors Corporation, Ford Motor Company, Chrysler, and the United Automobile Workers of America. Employees from the big banks and utility companies also joined. They all promised to work with members of the black community to heal the city. It seemed like a good idea, so I became an observer of the process.

Joseph L. Hudson, president of the Hudson-Webber Foundation, was the first chairman of the committee. In 2002, 35 years after the first meeting, Hudson was quoted in *The Detroit News* as saying, "We thought we'd find quick solutions to society's ills." Of course, there were no quick fixes in Detroit. In fact, I quickly left the committee because I found some of the same racism that sparked the riots still alive and kicking among some of the committee members.

I was a young guy in my early thirties, but I had been through a lot and seen the worst of the riot's tragedies. However, all I could do was sit there and watch a lot of bigwigs talk about how they were going to rebuild the city. Sure, they talked about how they were going to put hundreds of millions of dollars into new buildings. But when the heads of industry asked the unions to train more carpenters, plumbers, and electricians for the massive construction job, some of the union leaders basically said, "Do what you want, we're never going to hire blacks. We're just not going to do it in the automotive industry. You're trying to break the union; you're not trying to do anything good for anybody." With that, I said, "I'm moving somewhere, I'm going somewhere else. There is no hope for Detroit."

The New Detroit Committee later became known as New Detroit, Inc. The group continues to work toward racial equality and has had many successful initiatives. However, recent U.S. Census Bureau reports still identify Detroit as one of the most segregated cities in America. It is important to note that there were a lot of well-intentioned people on that first committee, but the attitudes of a few were enough to make me abandon hope for Detroit forever.

My Beginning in Diabetes Research

Once I decided to leave Detroit, I knew I wanted to do more research and expand my knowledge of endocrinology and metabolism. I had already finished one fellowship and spent an additional year teaching at Henry Ford Hospital. Those experiences influenced my decision to explore academic medicine, and I took a Fellowship position at the University of California Medical Center in San Francisco.

Talk about culture shock. I moved from riot-wracked Detroit to San Francisco in 1968 soon after the "summer of love." It was such a different environment. Detroit had hardened me to some degree and I didn't have that sunny optimism that many in San Francisco had. Plus, I was a kid who grew up on a farm and then went to schools where I wore a tie everyday of my life. The "free love" and "come as you are" mentality of the city was really new to me. But it didn't take long to get used to San Francisco. So much about the city appealed to me. It was, and is, a beautiful place. In a short time, California felt like home.

I learned so much at UC Med Center. During my first year, I became interested in diabetes treatment. It was the first time a medical professional came right out and told me that it was wrong to treat the disease with a high-fat diet. I still recall the moment like it was yesterday.

I met with my new chief, Peter Forsham, for the first time. This was the man who was going to be in charge of my professional life for the next two years. That fateful day, I nervously approached his secretary. She had more paper piled on her desk than anyone I had ever seen before. She said, "Oh yes, go in there and sit down. He'll be with you. He's on the phone right now."

I walked into an even smaller room, perhaps no bigger than six by eight feet with just enough room for his desk and a small couch. The office was crammed with even more papers than those on the secretary's desk. I sat down on the loveseat, which was legendary. All of the younger doctors referred to it as "The Famous Little Red Couch." So many had sat there before me, listening to Dr. Forsham dispense wisdom and advice. More than once, I was told, "When you talk to him, you will learn more in those few minutes sitting on that couch then you've ever learned before!"

I sat there for several minutes, watching this great man talking on the telephone to somebody. Without interrupting his conversation, he reached over and picked out a See's candy, popped it into his mouth, and ate it.

Dr. Forsham was a diabetic. How could he do this? I was stunned, to say the least! Then, before I even had time to consider the implications of his actions, he ate a second one! I looked at him, and he wasn't sweating. He wasn't having low blood sugar. He just looked like a regular guy enjoying a piece of candy.

When he picked up the third piece, I had a panicked mental dialogue with myself that went, *Oh my God, is he testing me? If so, what am I supposed to do? I can't grab the box out of his hands. Can I? No. That would be weird. Now what?*

Then, without skipping a word of his conversation, he reached over, picked up a vile of insulin from his top drawer, fished out a syringe, drew some insulin up, and shot it right through his pant leg. My head was spinning. Again, I thought, *What kind of test is this? I'm surely going to fail because I feel like I'm about to faint!*

He was breaking every single rule about dealing with diabetes. I knew that he had had diabetes since he was nine years old. But just how long had he been eating chocolate and shooting insulin through his pant leg? I was on the edge of that little red couch, wondering if every medical professional I had ever met was wrong, or if Dr. Forsham was just crazy. Or was I about to learn something incredible?

Dr. Forsham did not disappoint. He hung up the phone and turned to me with a pleasant smile. I had once heard him speak in Detroit and had been impressed, so as I shook his hand, I told him how much I admired his work. He warmly smiled again and said, "Well, I know you're here to work on adrenal disease because I see that you have been working on growth, and you probably want to continue with that. But since you're new and don't know how we work yet, I have another idea."

He told me about a grant the university had received to work on a new diabetes pill. It didn't have a name yet. It was only referred to by number. The drug, known under the name Glyburide, treats Type 2 (non-insulin dependent) diabetes by causing the pancreas to produce insulin, thus lowering blood sugar. In 1968, a German pharmaceutical company had just introduced the drug.

I listened to Dr. Forsham explain the medication. Then I thanked him for telling me about the project, but I said, "I'm not interested in diabetes research." He looked me straight in the eye and with much of the warmth in his voice gone, he asked, "Why not?" Again, I thought he was testing me. I replied, "Well the problem with diabetes is that I feel that no matter what we do, no matter how hard the patient tries, there seems to be little that can be done to keep them from the inevitable complications of the disease."

Dr. Forsham said, "Well it won't be long before you'll find out that you've got it all wrong. There's a better way to manage this illness. You'll see." Before I could protest, he said, "Now, let's get started. I need to tell you how to work on this project. I know you'll have ideas on how you would like to set it up, but the company has certain end points, so we'll have to follow much of their protocol. You'll get something very special out of this, much more than just your research results."

That is how I started working in the field of diabetes. Overall, the two years I spent working under Dr. Forsham were astounding. I learned more than I thought possible. I heard doctors discuss revolutionary treatment theories. Many of the medics at UCSF were so far ahead of their time that more traditional doctors would have surely called their work reckless. For instance, we would often have little meetings on Wednesday nights where

Nobel Prize winners from the university would speak to us. Most of them had retired, but they were still very sharp and full of new ideas.

There was one person, Royal Lee, DDS, whom I particularly remember because he correctly predicted the future. He was a Nobel Prize contender for synthesizing vitamins. During our talk, he made a comment about Vitamin E that has stuck with me ever since. He said, "I synthesized Vitamin E. I have no idea what it is, what it does, or what role it plays in human biology. But there are two things about it that you ought to remember. One is that for rats, it helps in their sexual development and abilities. Now, it's important to realize that there's no evidence that it will work for you." Our room, full of mostly young men and a few young women, burst out laughing.

Then he said something even more amazing. He told us, "Vitamin E is the most powerful antioxidant in nature. We don't know what that's good for right now. But someday you're going to know and it's going be extremely important." He was proven right. Antioxidants, including vitamin E, are critical to many of the body's functions and we now understand much more about how they work."

At UCSF Med Center, I also had the privilege of knowing another older gentleman, who wasn't a doctor or scholar, but a pioneer of sorts. When Joe was a kid back in the 1920s, he was given insulin. Before the discovery of insulin in 1921, nearly everyone diagnosed with Type 1 diabetes died within a few years. Of course, insulin didn't cure diabetes, but it was the first major step in the treatment of the disease. When I met him, Joe was a crusty, old guy who was still alive to tell great stories, thanks to the insulin shots he started receiving as a child. He could tell the most fascinating tales about being thrown in the back of a wagon and carried down to a funny place where he was told that they had a new thing that was going to make him better. Later, after I left UCSF, he became one of my patients.

The more time I spent at UCSF, the more I wished to specialize in diabetes. Diabetes challenged me because there were so many unknowns. Other endocrine illnesses could be worked on within the current knowledge. Diabetes was like a festering sore that never really got under control.

Now we know that people can prevent and even treat Type 2 diabetes with lifestyle changes. It takes effort to make those changes, but it can be done. Doctors need to educate patients and empower them to help themselves. Unfortunately, the knowledge that they need is still hard to access in a simple way.

C H A P T E R   5

Understanding Diabetes

There have been many changes in the field of diabetes since my days conducting research under Dr. Forsham at UCSF. We now know so much more about the causes and the treatments of the disease. To understand how far we've come in the battle I need to explain the basic facts of the disease.

Diabetes is the sixth leading cause of death in the United States. It is the main cause of kidney failure, limb amputations, and new onset blindness in adults. It is also one of the major causes of heart disease and stroke. There is no known cure.

Diabetes presents many symptoms and complications, all of which involve problems with the body's insulin production and usage. Insulin is a hormone that is made in the pancreas and regulates the amount of glucose that reaches the cells throughout the body. Glucose is the main sugar circulating through the blood and a major source of energy. Most of the food we eat each day is broken down into glucose. People with diabetes do not make enough insulin, improperly use the insulin they produce, or both. This causes too much glucose to accumulate in the blood, causing major problems throughout the body.

Some of the most common symptoms of diabetes

include:

- Frequent urination
- Weariness
- Increased thirst, hunger, or both
- Sudden weight loss
- Blurred vision
- Very dry skin
- Tingling or numbness in the hands or feet

Types of Diabetes

Type 1 Diabetes

Type 1 diabetes, previously called juvenile diabetes or insulin-dependent diabetes mellitus, develops quickly and the symptoms are obvious. Most people contract this form of diabetes as children or teenagers. The body's immune system destroys pancreatic beta cells, which are the only cells in the body that make insulin. Without enough beta cells to make insulin, blood glucose levels dramatically rise, causing a condition called hyperglycemia. Patients with Type 1 diabetes require insulin injections to maintain their health.

Often, Type 1 diabetics experience a honeymoon period after the disease is diagnosed. Symptoms disappear and it seems like the body has conquered the disease. This period can last for a few months or as long as a year. During this time, the patient may not require insulin. Eventually, the patient will lose most, if not all, of their insulin-producing cells and will have to depend on insulin, eventually becoming totally dependent on insulin injections.

People with Type 1 diabetes have a life expectancy 15 years less than someone without the disease. It is still not entirely clear what causes Type 1 diabetes, but some risk factors include genetics, autoimmune disorders, and environmental influences. Less than 10% of the people with diabetes have Type 1 diabetes.

Type 2 Diabetes

Type 2 diabetes is more common and used to be known as non-insulin-dependent diabetes or adult-onset diabetes. Unlike Type 1 diabetes, this disease develops slowly over time and symptoms are less severe. In fact, many people do not notice any symptoms and are surprised when their doctors inform them that they have diabetes. Experts estimate that nearly 20 million Americans may have Type 2 diabetes, but many of them don't even know it.

Type 2 diabetes begins with a problem called insulin resistance. In that state, insulin cannot properly move glucose to the cells that need it. The body tries to compensate by making more insulin. However, the pancreas can only keep up the elevated pace of insulin production for so long. Over time, the pancreas becomes less effective and may eventually wear out. With a decreased amount of insulin in circulation, glucose levels rise after eating a meal. Left untreated, the condition continues to worsen and beta cells begin to die. Over time, glucose levels remain too high even between meals.

Risk factors of Type 2 diabetes include:

- Obesity

- Age beyond 45 years

- Family history of the disease

- A previous occurrence of gestational diabetes, or a pregnancy resulting in a baby weighing more than nine pounds

- Ethnicity: African-Americans, Hispanic/Latino Americans, American Indians, Asian-Americans, and Pacific Islanders have an increased risk of developing Type 2 diabetes

- High blood pressure

- Lack of exercise

- HDL cholesterol level of 35 or lower or a triglyceride level of 250 or higher

Gestational Diabetes

Gestational diabetes is a form of Type 2 diabetes that only affects pregnant women. About 5% of expectant mothers will develop the disease in their third trimester of pregnancy. Fortunately, gestational diabetes is generally temporary, but it can cause serious problems. Risk factors include obesity and a family history of the disease. Like Type 2 diabetes, Hispanic, American Indian, African-American, and Asian-American women are more prone to developing it. Women who have had gestational diabetes have a higher chance of developing Type 2 diabetes in the decade after their pregnancies.

Other Factors

In about 1% of cases, diabetes occurs as a result of other factors. Diseases that affect the pancreas, including pancreatitis, can spark the onset of diabetes. Some drugs, including beta-blockers and corticosteroids, can temporarily cause the disease. In rarer cases, malnutrition and infection can also cause diabetes.

Effects and Complications of Diabetes

Many people still think diabetes is a disease about sugar. This is such a big misconception that I often want to scream from the rooftops, "IT'S NOT THE SUGAR! IT'S THE COMPLICATIONS!" No one dies from too much sugar anymore. They die of complications caused by the problems that arise when they have problems with glucose regulation. Diabetics die of heart disease and secondary metabolic conditions, not sugar intake.

Neuropathy is one of the major complications of diabetics. It strikes in many forms and can be painful and debilitating. Neuropathy occurs when nerves fail to carry information to and from the brain and spinal cord. There are two main types of neuropathy, each affecting different types of nerve cells. One is called peripheral neuropathy, which affects the nerves that control sensation in the body. It can cause both pain and the inability to feel pain. Loss of sensation, or lack of pain reception, is especially dangerous because people with neuropathy can hurt themselves without knowing it.

The other type of neuropathy is autonomic neuropathy. It affects nerves that control various organs, such as your stomach or urinary tract. Maintaining blood glucose levels can control both types of neuropathy. With vigilant monitoring, the chance of developing nerve damage is greatly reduced.

The human eye is also very vulnerable to the effects of diabetes. Many people experience blurred vision in the early stages of the disease. The most serious eye problem that can occur with diabetes is damage to the retina, the thin, light-sensitive lining in the back of your eye. This damage occurs to small blood vessels in the retina, which are easily harmed by high blood glucose levels. Complete blindness is rare if retinopathy is diagnosed early and treated promptly.

Diabetics often suffer from kidney failure. This is a silent problem, meaning its complications can be symptomless until they are in their advanced states. Over a period of time, high blood glucose damages the filtering systems in the kidneys, hindering their ability to pass waste out through the urine. Once this damage occurs, it can't be repaired. However, screening tests and medical treatment can slow the damage and prevent end-stage renal failure that requires kidney transplant or dialysis.

Peripheral vascular disease is a complication of diabetes. It is impaired circulation that can, if left unchecked, lead to gangrene, non-healing foot wounds, and amputation. It is caused by the build-up of cholesterol in the blood vessels of the lower extremities.

Poorly controlled diabetes can also lead to skin problems. Excessively dry skin occurs due to dehydration from high blood glucose, and "shin spots" can develop on the front of the legs (these are harmless and are nothing to worry about). Orange-yellow fatty plaques may also appear around the eyes or on the shins or elbows.

Perhaps the most troubling problem commonly

experienced by diabetics is advanced atherosclerosis, which involves the build-up of plaque deposits in the blood vessels. It can cause hardening of the arteries, heart attack, or stroke. Researchers have found that a cardiovascular disease is a chief cause of death in people whose diabetes developed after age 30.

Until recently, cause of death was often stated as hardening of the arteries. However, somewhere in the list of problems, diabetes would be listed. In reality, diabetes was the cause of most, if not all, of the health problems that caused death. This lack of clarity has caused national statistics on disease to be somewhat misrepresented. The American public has thought that heart disease is our foremost health problem. People don't realize that diabetes is involved in many cases of heart disease. As this becomes more generally known, endocrinologists can have more success in treating the cause and the complications. The general population also needs to know this. The complications of diabetes can occur as early as seven years before the diagnosis of the disease. Below is a partial list of the complications and what you can do to check for them:

Coronary Heart Disease

- Review the laboratory results
- Check the long arteries in the legs for atherosclerosis

Peripheral and Autonomic Neuropathy (50% of patients with a diabetic diagnosis experience this)

- Measure sensation (nerve activity)

• Measure response (nerve function)

Blood Pressure Elevation

• Check blood pressure

Insulin Resistance

• Decrease weight by various means

• Exercise regularly, within achievable limits

• Take medication to "break" insulin resistance

Laboratory Results: a patient can delay or prevent the presence of diabetes by assessing risk factors and altering them. Have the following laboratory tests performed:

• HbA1c, Fructosamine

• Cholesterol (lipid) patterns

• Highly sensitive C-reactive protein

• Microalbumin

• GAD antibodies (for Type 1)

• Three-day glucose monitor-checks glucose every 10 seconds

• Homocysteine

Treatment Options

Although the complications of diabetes can be very serious and even deadly, they can be largely prevented. Studies indicate that patients with both Type 1 and Type 2 diabetes can maintain their health if they keep blood glucose levels in check. Type 1 diabetics must take insulin. If they don't, they face certain death. For Type 2 diabetics, successful treatment depends on many factors, including the individual's commitment to lifestyle choices that are necessary to maintain good health.

The most common and effective therapies for Type 2 diabetes include sticking to a healthy diet, exercise, and blood glucose testing. Diabetics must monitor their blood glucose levels carefully to make sure the amount of insulin is balanced with their food consumption and physical exertion. Many Type 2 diabetics can keep their blood glucose levels in an acceptable range without taking medication. This is largely dependent on whether they stay at a healthy weight and follow a diabetic diet.

However, it is important to realize that even if Type 2 diabetics can keep their disease under control with diet and exercise, they still have diabetes. The disease never goes away. It requires constant monitoring. If a patient gains weight, stops exercising, or even overeats at a meal, their blood glucose levels will rise. Stress can also increase the severity of the disease. Some people with Type 2 diabetes will have to take oral medication, insulin injections, or both to maintain proper glucose levels, even when keeping to a strict diet and exercise plan. This is especially common as patients grow older. I have seen many patients who have had satisfactory blood glucose levels for much of their adult life discover that their insulin production has decreased over time, and their insulin resistance has increased.

Because diabetes is a disease that can fluctuate, patients must continue to check their blood glucose levels, even when they experience no symptoms. Although acceptable ranges will vary slightly among individuals, most patients should keep their plasma blood glucose below 140 mg/dl before eating and 180 mg/dl two hours after eating. Sometimes patients will notice a spike. However, if levels remain high for more than a few days, it is important to notify a doctor because current treatment plans may no longer be effective.

In addition to self-monitoring, physicians recommend that patients undergo a hemoglobin A1c test two to four times a year. This test, which is most commonly referred to as an A1c, measures the average blood sugar over the past two to three months. It is the most widely used test to measure a person's overall diabetes control. Physicians will look to see that the results stay at 7.0 or lower. If the test comes back with an 8.0 or higher, generally it is time to explore new treatment options.

New Research and Drug Therapies

Until fairly recently, sulfonylureas were the only types of medication available for treating Type 2 diabetes. Sulfonylureas work by stimulating the pancreas to make more insulin. This class of drugs includes DiaBeta (glyburide), Diabinese (chlorpropamide), and Orinase (tolbutamide), along with several others. Non-sulfonylureas also help the pancreas produce more insulin, but through a slightly different reaction. The most common non-sulfonylurea is metformin.

In the past few years, new medications have become available, expanding the treatment options for Type 2 diabetics. These drugs are different from previous drugs because, instead of forcing the body to make more insulin, they make the body more sensitive to the effects of the insulin it is already producing. Insulin sensitizers include the thiazolidinediones Actos (pioglitazone) and Avandia (rosiglitazone).

Some patients do well when taking alpha-glucosidase inhibitors. These so-called "starch blockers" slow the intestinal absorption of the carbohydrates eaten. This process lessens the spikes in blood glucose levels in the bloodstream. Examples of these drugs include Glyset (miglitol) and Precose (acarbose).

In March 2005, I started using the new injectable drug, Symlin, in my patients. The FDA approved the drug to help control blood glucose levels in people with both Type 1 and Type 2 diabetes. It has been used primarily in patients who have not done well on insulin therapy. Symlin is a synthetic version of the hormone, amylin, which is secreted along with insulin. Used with insulin, Symlin works to lower blood sugar for three hours after a meal. My patients have done well on Symlin, although some people did gain a few pounds while on the drug.

The drug I am most excited about right now is Byetta. It is a sister drug to Symlin, and they both came out at the same time. I have reason to believe that Byetta may have the power to completely reverse diabetes. The process of bringing Byetta to the market has taken a long time, and there have been serious setbacks. Although we've known that the drug has amazing potential, it also carries risks. Although the FDA trials were ok, Byetta might have led to serious low blood glucose. Instead of banning its use, the FDA carefully weighed Byetta's enormous benefits. In order to further explore its usage, the government decided to release the drug to only about 80 doctors in the United States. I was fortunate enough to be included in the program. The FDA basically left it to the doctors to figure out how it can be used to help, not harm. For three months, Company officials came to my office everyday to monitor my work and the progress of my patients.

My patients have done so well on Byetta that I think it could be the next miracle drug. It allows the body to re-grow cells that are dying due to diabetes. In order to reduce the risks associated with the drug, I've adapted its usage in my practice. The success has been striking. Byetta became available to the general population in June of 2005. Used correctly, this drug could dramatically improve the health of diabetics.

In addition to Byetta and Symlin, there are other new drugs under development that may increase treatment options. A choice of medications is important since all drugs may not have the same effect on everyone. Many times, drugs that control blood glucose in one patient will be completely ineffective in another patient. Finding the right medication is often achieved through experimentation. Even then, a patient may find that the right drug will stop working effectively over time. In the past, when a drug option became ineffective, the patient would most likely have to start using insulin. Today new drugs on the market allow endocrinologists to try different drug approaches until blood glucose levels are brought under control.

Metabolic X Syndrome

Research is also now underway to treat obesity more effectively by discovering more about Metabolic X Syndrome. This could reduce the incidence of diabetes. Scientists at Joslin Diabetes Center in Boston have discovered genes that cause the growth of "brown fat." Most of us are familiar with white fat, which is the fat stored for use as energy. It's what we burn off through diet and exercise. Brown fat is used to generate heat and burn calories. Babies are born with brown fat in their necks, which helps them stay warm. Brown fat usually disappears by the time we become adults.

Scientists are now trying to figure out how to help adults reduce brown fat, which would reduce insulin resistance. If more is learned about the genes that control the production of brown fat cells, scientists may be able to help people who are genetically predisposed to obesity.

CHAPTER 6

Dangerous Diets

As a child, I enjoyed all of the food that was readily available on our farm. I've mentioned the mountains of food that the hired men would plow through. It was a sight to see! The men would load their plates high with mashed potatoes, gravy, meat, and vegetables. They would top it all off with two or three types of pie. I loved eating right along with them. Never once did I think about the connection between what I ate and the health of my body.

Today, we are concerned that the typical American diet is causing all types of diseases, including diabetes. However, the farm hands were not fat men. In fact, they were lean. Their tremendously physical work forced their bodies to burn every calorie they consumed. The men who worked in our community didn't have combines; they had to use thrashers. The invention of combines reduced the physical labor required for harvesting crops. Life on the farms of today is still tough, but farmers don't work the same way. Unfortunately, as the amount of physical activity needed from America's workforce has declined, waistlines have increased. Too many Americans now live sedentary lives sitting behind desks all day, but they still eat like those farm hands.

Sometimes cultural practices have an impact. I have

Mexican patients who have considered it appropriate to consume many tortillas, even though they get little physical exercise. This norm is not healthy. Diabetes rates have increased greatly in the Mexican-American community, largely because of high-calorie diets containing carbohydrates and fats.

There is societal pressure to eat. It begins with parents who encourage their children to eat more so they will become "big and strong." Throughout our childhood, we are rewarded for a job well done with cookies or ice cream. There is nothing wrong with giving a child a special treat, but rewarding kids with food can lead to a habit of eating for emotional reasons. I have many patients who must resist the urge to reach for chocolate when they are sad or a bag of chips when they are bored. It is simply what they have always done.

Poor dietary choices have had a devastating effect on our health. More than two-thirds of American adults are now overweight, and half of those are obese. Some studies suggest that eight out of ten Americans should lose some weight for optimal health, even if they are not considered overweight by medical standards. Excess weight increases your chances of getting diabetes, heart disease, some types of cancer, strokes, and other conditions.

While we spend billions of dollars a year on diet books, exercise equipment, and weight loss supplements, the problem with obesity in our country is getting worse. According to the federal government, in 1980, 46 percent of American adults were overweight. In 2000, the number had jumped to more than 64 percent! As early as 1988, former Surgeon General C. Everett Koop reported that a poor diet was the leading preventable contributor to premature death in the U.S.

It is not just adults who are getting fatter. Childhood obesity in the United States is increasing at an astonishing rate. Nearly 15 percent of kids are overweight. Unless we prevent this, today's children will be the first generation of Americans to have a shorter life span and decreased health expectancy. It used to be rare to hear of kids with Type 2 diabetes, but we are seeing frequent cases of it today as more and more children become overweight.

In a study commissioned by the Gerber Products Co., it was discovered that many American children under the age of two already have the same bad eating habits as their parents. Children between the ages of one and two only need about 950 calories a day, but in the study, the median intake of calories was 1,220. That is 30 percent more calories than recommended.

In the survey of the eating habits of 3,000 children, about a third of children under the age of two ate no fruits or vegetables on that day. Among the children who did eat vegetables, French fries were the most common selection. Hot dogs, sausage and bacon were at the top of the list of foods most consumed. Sixty percent of the parents reported that their toddlers ate dessert or candy at least once a day. All of these findings are startling because lifelong food preferences are commonly thought to be shaped between the ages of two and three. It certainly doesn't look good for the future health of these young children if they already downing large quantities fatty meats and soft drinks.

Sugar vs. Complex Carbs

Whether you have diabetes or want to prevent it, the recommended diets are similar. Research has lead to new and helpful conclusions about how to eat for optimal health, but most people are not yet benefiting from this knowledge. The idea is to maintain an eating plan to keep blood glucose levels under control. You can make eating this way very complicated or very simple. I prefer to keep it simple. First, let's talk about sugar.

Until about seven ago, diabetics were told not to eat simple sugar but to consume more complex carbohydrates, like those contained in brown rice or whole-grain cereal. While that's not bad advice, it is not complete advice. People with diabetes can include some sugar in their diets and keep their blood glucose levels under control. The goal is to keep track of the total grams of carbohydrates being consumed during the day and to not overload on carbs at any one meal or snack. Your dietician should help you figure out how many carbs you can safely consume in a day.

Unlike in the past, there are no longer "banned" foods for diabetics. But, you should still use common sense. Even a non-diabetic should not get all of their daily carbs from ice cream! Everyone needs the nutrients and fiber that come from eating healthy carbs obtained from fruits, vegetables, and whole grains.

Tips for Healthy Eating

Most of us, including diabetics, would be well-served to reduce portion sizes and the amount of fat we eat. When you do eat, make sure you are getting a variety of unprocessed, nutritious foods. Here are some guidelines to follow:

- Avoid saturated fats found in butter, solid shortening, and palm and coconut oil.

- Limit red meat.

- Buy only nonfat or low-fat dairy products.

- Do not fry foods. Switch to baking, broiling, or poaching. You can also sauté food with some cooking spray in a nonstick pan.

- Stay away from refined sugar. Sweets provide calories but no nutritional value.

- Eliminate most white flour. Like sugar, refined grains provide empty calories and no fiber. Choose whole grains, like whole wheat, brown rice, barley, and oats.

- Reduce salt intake. It can raise your blood pressure.

- Learn to read food labels so you can detect fat, sugar, and salt in foods.

- Don't skip meals. If you know you are going to miss a meal, have a snack ready. This will help keep your blood sugar in balance.

- Limit alcohol. If you must have a drink, enjoy it with food so it has less effect on the blood sugar.

These tips are easier to follow at home than in a restaurant. Unfortunately, Americans are now eating more meals at restaurants, where portions are getting bigger. The Center for Science in the Public Interest estimates that the typical restaurant meal contains about 1,000 calories, without counting appetizers and desserts. Add a fried starter and gooey dessert to your meal and you're well above 2,000 calories. Catherine Reade, MS, RD has provided some strategies to follow when dining out:

(Reproduced with permission of IDEA Health & Fitness Association, www.IDEAfit.com.)

- Start each meal with a large glass of water. Ask for refills throughout the meal. Water fills you up without adding any calories (plus it's free).

- Balance your food budget. If you know you will be having beefsteak for dinner, choose lighter fare for lunch.

- Choose a restaurant that prepares low-fat fare and preplan your menu choices before you arrive. Or call ahead to make sure the establishment has what you desire.

- Be an aggressive diner. Before ordering, ask how the food selections are prepared and make special requests for low-fat meals.

- Order the smallest size. Even though the biggest meal portions appear to give you the best value, resist and opt for the smallest burger or the plain grilled chicken sandwich.

- When in doubt, order simple dishes. Foods like grilled halibut, steamed vegetables, and a plain baked potato are all low-fat choices.

- Order salad dressings and sauces on the side. Rather than the restaurant's kitchen heaping dressings and sauces on your meal, this strategy lets you control the amount of fat you ingest.

- Avoid French fries. Like all fried foods, French fries contain excessive amounts of fat. On rare occasions when you must indulge yourself, order the smallest size.

- Relish your favorite foods. If you adore crusty bread, go for it, but round out your meal with a salad and fruit. If you have your heart set on a large entrée, skip the appetizers and the bread and butter.

- Share an order or take half home. When your meal arrives, ask for a take-out box and immediately put away half of your meal before you start. Better yet, ask for a half-portion at a reduced rate.

- Start meals with a fruit or vegetable. These fiber-filled foods will be filling and leave less room for calorie-dense food.

Grazing

I also recommend forgetting the "three square meals" rule. It is better to "graze" throughout the day. When you graze you consume very small meals and snacks, without ever letting too much time pass between eating. By eating this way, there is never a big load placed on the already-impaired pancreas, allowing for a more sustained and lowered calorie release. Often diabetics use medications to slow the absorption of calories. By eating smaller meals throughout the day, these medications become largely unnecessary.

Diabetics need to be very consistent about the calories they consume each day. A balance should be achieved between diet and exercise. If you eat more than normal, you have to be prepared for more activity or, in some cases, insulin. Just how many calories should you take in? There is no one answer to that question. Each individual's dietary requirements are unique.

I usually send a new diabetic patient to a dietician. It is important that they spend time with a professional structuring an appropriate diet. The amount you eat depends on many factors, including weight, height, and medical condition. Don't just follow printed "diabetic diets." I also tell my patients not to be influenced by the latest popular diet. People should eat what works best for their bodies. With the help of your dietician, come up with a plan that makes you feel physically at your best.

Thanks in large part to my wife, I am eating healthier. My dinner last night was pretty typical for our household. I had salmon, beans, and a small glass of wine. I was full and felt satisfied. I had eaten vegetables and fruit throughout the day, so I knew that I had done a good job covering my nutritional needs.

Everyone has his or her weaknesses when it comes to food. I love hamburgers and I may even eat one tonight. However, hamburgers are only an occasional treat for me. My wife and I choose to emphasize vegetables in our diet and focus on the eating foods we enjoy that are also good for us.

The Importance of Exercise

I have loved running since I was a teenager. I find there is no better way for me to reduce stress. There is something so calming about the repetitive motion of my feet hitting the pavement. After my workout, I love experiencing the so-called "runner's high" when endorphins are shooting through my body. It is an incredible, natural mood elevator. Of course, I also run to keep myself healthy. Next to diet, exercise is most important.

As a society, we spend too much of our time sitting down. When I talk to new patients, I often find that they work all day behind a desk and then come home and relax by sitting on the couch watching television. This may be considered normal today, but it is proving deadly! A poor diet, combined with a sedentary lifestyle, dramatically increases the risk of diabetes, heart disease, and many forms of cancer.

Our bodies are built for activity. Throughout history, humans have had to move to stay alive. Covering basic needs required physical work. That's not the case any more and Americans are paying for it. Almost all modern inventions, including automobiles and computers, have been designed to reduce physical activity. Thanks to the car, we no longer need to walk to do our errands. Increasingly, we don't even need to walk to our garages to get our cars. All of our errands, including our banking and shopping, can be done over the Internet.

When I recommend an exercise program to my new patients, many of them look at me with a mix of fear and dread. The idea of incorporating more physical activity into their day seems difficult to them. I assure them that just making small changes in their daily routine can have major benefits.

Exercise has so many positive effects on your body. Here's some of what you can expect when you get moving:

- Reduced risk of many diseases, including diabetes, cancer, and osteoporosis
- Reduced body fat
- Increased muscle mass that allows the body to look and function better
- Improved circulation
- Lower blood pressure
- Boosted immunity
- Less stress
- A positive impact on mood and feelings of self-worth
- Higher sex drive
- Better skin tone
- Increased energy levels and less fatigue

Exercise is especially important to people with diabetes. When you exercise, the body uses glucose for as this fuel is burned. Physical activity also triggers a reaction in your body that allows glucose to enter your cells, where it is properly utilized.

There are misconceptions about exercise. First, start now, at any age or time, as it is never too late to start. Even if you have been inactive for years, exercise will immediately start improving your health. You don't have to be an athlete or already be in good shape to workout. Many of the most beneficial exercises require no special ability. You don't need to go to a gym, lift heavy weights, buy expensive equipment, or start playing sports to incorporate exercise into your life. You just need to move! Walking, dancing, and gardening all count as physical activity. The key is to be consistently active. You will not reach your fitness potential by mowing the grass once a week or taking an occasional stroll around the neighborhood. The goal should be to fit in at least 30 minutes of exercise on most days of the week.

If you have been inactive for a while, it can be tough to start an exercise program. Therefore, I recommend beginning slowly with simple activities like walking. However, to get the maximum benefits from exercise, you'll eventually want to do more. There are three components of physical fitness and each one is equally important for good health.

Aerobic Exercise is any activity that keeps your heart rate up for an extended period of time. Examples of aerobic exercise include walking and jogging, swimming, dancing, and skating. There are also many types of equipment designed for aerobic conditioning, such as equipment designed for aerobic conditioning, such as treadmills, stair machines, and elliptical trainers. Aerobic exercise strengthens your cardiovascular system, which is the functioning of your heart and lungs. During aerobic exercise, your heart and lungs have to work harder to take oxygen from the air and supply it to all of the cells in your body. With continued aerobic exercise, your cardiovascular system grows stronger and more efficient.

Aerobic exercise burns fat, helping you lose weight. During aerobic exercise, you burn up to 20 times more calories than when you are just sitting in front of the television. Over time, all of that calorie burning can add up to substantial weight loss. Additionally, aerobic activity lowers your levels of bad cholesterol and increases bone strength.

Ideally, you should try to fit in at least 20 to 30 minutes of aerobic exercise three to five times a week. If you are just starting out, go slowly and do only what you can comfortably manage. Perhaps that means only a five-minute walk. That's fine. Walk for five minutes. Next week, aim for seven minutes. Gradually, you'll build up strength and endurance until you are able to reach your goals.

For people who have never exercised regularly, I strongly recommend walking. Not only it is a great form of aerobic exercise, it is simple, free, and requires no special equipment except for sturdy shoes. Recently, there have been several studies showing that taking 10,000 steps a day can bring significant health benefits, including a reduced risk of heart disease. That is about four miles, average person only walks only 900 to 3,000 steps per day.

You can track the number of steps you take in a day with a pedometer attached to your belt. Pedometers can be a fun way to chart your progress. However, you can also just try to incorporate more walking into your everyday tasks. Some good ways include:

- Take a walk before work or during your lunch break.

- Stop wasting time looking for a parking space. You'll almost always find a space at the farthest end of the lot. Park there and walk.

- Use the stairs whenever possible.

- Ask your significant other to take a nightly walk with you. You'll be able to spend quality time together while doing something that is good for both of you.

To enjoy the benefits of a well-rounded exercise program, you'll eventually have to do more than just walk, but it's a good start!

Strength Training is essential to building and maintaining lean muscle mass. This type of activity is also called anaerobic exercise, which involves short bursts of energy, followed by a period of rest. Anaerobic means "without air" because these intense bursts of power are so short, oxygen does not have time to travel to the muscles. Your muscles quickly fatigue during anaerobic exercise. For example, you may be able to walk for 20 minutes, but you could not (and should not) lift and lower a heavy weight continuously for that long.

weight continuously for that long.

Muscle gains strength by performing more exertion than it is used to. Lifting weights, using stretch tubing and bands, and Nautilus equipment are all good ways to strength train. There are also plenty of strength-training exercises that require absolutely no equipment, including push-ups, sit-ups, and squats.

There is a misconception that strength training is performed for the purpose of building huge muscles. Strength training is for everyone, no matter the age or physical condition. There is no better way to reverse the aging process. Like aerobic exercise, anaerobic activity can lower your chance of developing diabetes, heart disease, cancer, and osteoporosis. However, carefully designed strength-training programs also reduce some forms of chronic pain such as arthritis, and make daily tasks much easier. When you work against resistance, you build muscle, which makes you better able to do all kinds of things, from lifting a bag of groceries to getting out of chair.

Some women are afraid to strength train because they don't want to build bulky muscles. This is an unfounded fear. The vast majority of women do not have the hormones necessary to build large muscles. It is just not possible, unless they are taking steroids. However, strength training will help people of both sexes achieve toned, slimmer bodies. The advantage of building muscle is that it forces your body to burn more calories throughout the day by revving up your metabolism, even when you are not exercising. Every pound of muscle gained uses up 50 extra calories a day, which translates into less fat more calories at all times, including when you are just sitting on the couch!

Strive to fit in at least two strength-training workouts each week. There are many great ways to strength train. No matter which method you choose, select exercises for all of the major muscle groups. The major muscle groups include your chest, arms, back, abdominals, and legs. Beginners can benefit greatly from taking part in group strength-training exercise classes. You can also hire a personal trainer to teach you proper exercise form. If you are not sure how to get started, ask your health care professional for help. He or she should be able to give you several options.

Flexibility is the most overlooked form of physical fitness. When you hear people talking about their workouts, they might mention how far they've walked or how much they were able to lift, but they almost never talk about how far they could reach. Increasing your body's ability to bend, twist, and reach will help you in just about every physical activity, from picking something off the floor to washing your back. Increasing your flexibility through stretching will help you be more limber and coordinated and greatly reduce your chance of injury.

Increased flexibility improves the daily aches and pains. So many times, what people mistake for the pains of "getting old" is really just a loss in flexibility. Tight muscles can make you hurt in all kinds of unexpected places. I have talked to many patients who suffer from low back pain. Often, they really are suffering from not being limber. For example, if you sit all day at a desk, computer, or behind the wheel of a car, the muscles in your hips will tighten. At the same time, the muscles in your buttocks will get too loose. This creates a major imbalance throughout the pelvic region. What seems like low back pain may come from a loss of flexibility in the hips. If you think you need pain medication, you might actually benefit more from a good stretch.

When you stretch your muscles, go slowly and do not stretch to the point of pain. You will experience a mild discomfort, but stretching should not hurt. Focus on static stretching, which means no bouncing. Even though we didn't know it at the time, those fast toe touches we used to do in gym class were a bad idea. That kind of quick stretching becomes even worse for us as we age and become less limber, making us more susceptible to injury. Hold each stretch for about 30 seconds while taking nice, deep breaths.

You should try to stretch for at least a total of 30 minutes a week. Start by stretching the muscles you have worked after every aerobic and strength training workout. Flexibility training can also be a workout of its own. Tai chi, yoga, and Pilates are all physical activities that focus on elongating the body.

Any exercise program requires a focus on proper form. Diabetics need to be extra careful because exercise can cause blood sugar to drop too low, causing hypoglycemia. Many diabetics are advised to carry glucose gel or tablets when exercising.

Even though you might need to take special precautions due to your medical condition, you should not avoid physical activity. People often cite their illness as an excuse to not exercise. I have diabetic patients who are policemen, scuba divers, exercise instructors, and even bungee jumpers. While I am not suggesting you start bungee jumping, diabetes should not place limits on what you can do. Move out of the mindset that diabetes has to alter your exercise, fun, and enjoyment.

I'd like to share a 2002 government study called the Diabetes Prevention Program which further demonstrated the power of exercise and a healthy diet. The research showed that people at risk for Type 2 diabetes could delay the onset of the disease or even prevent it with a simple regimen of moderate diet and exercise. The research also confirmed that the diabetes drug, Glucophage, could reduce the risk, but not as effectively as diet and exercise. Physical activity worked better than the drugs!

The study used volunteers who were considered to be at high risk for developing diabetes because they had a condition called impaired glucose tolerance. Impaired glucose tolerance is one of the precursors to Type 2 diabetes. In the study, participants who lost just 5% to 7% of their weight reduced the occurrence of Type 2 diabetes by 58%. People who were over the age of 60 reduced their risk by 71%! The research subjects achieved the weight loss by walking for about 30 minutes a day, five days a week and lowering the amount of calories and fat they consumed. The participants who took the drug had only a 31% lower incidence of developing the disease.

Glucophage and the lifestyle changes both lowered

blood glucose levels when fasting, but exercise was much more effective at lowering glucose levels two hours after a sugary drink. That is important because it means those who followed a diet and exercise program were able to actually reverse their impaired glucose tolerance.

Starting a diet and exercise program can seem overwhelming. Some patients tell me, "It's too hard!" I tell them, "Well, it's a lot easier than the complications you will be facing if you continue down your current path." Usually when my patients start seeing the benefits of their new, healthier lifestyles, they are motivated to continue their efforts. There is nothing more empowering than taking control of your health.

CHAPTER 7

Nutritional Supplements

My entire approach to practicing medicine changed when I was thirty-seven years old. I was diagnosed with generalized atherosclerosis, a threat of atherosclerotic heart disease. Atherosclerotic heart disease is the underlying cause of heart attacks and one of the main causes of congestive heart failure. It starts early in life, as cholesterol plaque builds up in the arteries of the heart and brain. Such build-up can increase the risk of heart attacks and strokes. The condition silently worsens with age. Although a family history of heart disease can make you more likely to develop the disease, smoking, diabetes, high cholesterol, and hypertension are all major contributing factors. In my case, I probably inherited the same heart disease that led to my father's stroke.

When I became aware of my condition, I thought, "This is it. I'm a doctor. I know what can happen here. I'm going to do something." But what was there to do? I knew that there was nothing in the framework of existing medicine that would adequately help me. Prescription drugs alone wouldn't do it.

In a moment of clarity, I said, "Okay. I'm not just a doctor. I am a metabolic specialist. If anybody can do this, I can. I've got to look at the way I live my entire life. Are some of my habits harming me? What am I doing that is good for me? Am I getting enough exercise?" So many variables ran through my head. I decided that I would give myself a total assessment and rid myself of the disease. And that is exactly what I did, even though almost no one at the time thought such a thing was possible.

L-arginine

I was diagnosed with atherosclerotic heart disease after a CAT scan of my stomach showed that I had calcification of the arteries. I started researching my condition by talking to colleagues and reading about new studies. That's how I found out about experiments that indicated l-arginine could be a powerful weapon against heart disease.

Arginine, which is an amino acid, is a protein that benefits the body in a myriad of ways. Discovered in 1895, arginine plays an important part in cell division, boosting immunity, healing wounds, and the secretion of hormones. When your body is under attack from infections or wounds, it burns through arginine quickly, so hospitals often give the supplement, l-arginine, to patients to speed recovery. In 1998, the Nobel Prize was awarded to three American scientists for their discovery in the role that arginine plays in the production of nitric oxide in the body. Nitric oxide is a dilator, meaning it helps the arteries relax and grow larger.

In 1991, I started taking 500mg of l-arginine twice a day. This was a very low dosage, so I wasn't sure it would have a measurable affect on my condition. After taking l-arginine for a while, I went to see the same radiologist for another CAT scan. We were both stunned by the results. The radiologist said to me, "How did you do this? You have gotten rid of all of the build-up in your arteries. You have reversed your condition. That's not possible!"

Thrilled and surprised by the CAT scan, I went for more tests, including a heart scan, to see how much atherosclerosis was affecting my heart. The heart scan came back as a zero, meaning I had no measurable atherosclerosis! My father had suffered a stroke in his forties and died in his early fifties from the same disease I had just reversed in myself.

Now that I had incorporated l-arginine into my life, I decided it was time to introduce it into my professional practice. The results have been nothing short of miraculous. In 1991, 30% of my diabetic patients ended up seeing a cardiologist for bypass procedures. I started routinely recommending l-arginine. In just nine short years, less than 1% of my patients needed to see a cardiologist for any reason. Since 1991, my practice has not had one patient suffer from a heart attack or stroke. It gives me great satisfaction to report that we have virtually reversed all heart disease, even in the patients who have other diabetes-related problems. We have always heard that you can't make progress in treating heart disease in diabetics until the patient has complete control over their blood glucose levels. That's obviously not true!

One of my friends and colleagues is a well-respected cardiologist. I used to refer a lot of patients to him. Recently, he said to me, "Did I do something to offend you? I've noticed that you no longer send patients to me." I said, "It's not you. I'm not sending my patients to anyone. They don't need cardiologists because we are reversing their heart disease!"

Arginine affects the entire vascular system. Because it makes arteries relax, blood flows better throughout the body. It also has had an unexpected, positive impact on plaque build up. Researchers have discovered that arginine therapy can reduce LDL, or "bad", cholesterol but does not reduce HDL, or "good", cholesterol. Medical professionals used to think that plaque would accumulate in the arteries until it completely closed them off. That's not correct. We now know that as plaque gets bigger, it becomes unstable and causes little breaks, or cuts, in the artery. The cuts then clot to stop the bleeding. This is dangerous. You obviously do not want clotting in your arteries. The clots also start a cascading effect of coagulation within the vascular system. Tiny clots begin to form in the brain, lungs, and other areas. Several studies have concluded that, in people with high cholesterol, l-arginine reduces the risk of blood platelets clumping, therefore lessening the chance of stroke and heart attacks.

There is good reason to believe that l-arginine can relieve hypertension by restoring blood pressure. In 1998, Italian researchers reported that daily doses of arginine reduced systolic blood pressure. This is major news for many reasons, not the least of which is that it could allow people to cut back on their prescription blood pressure medications, therefore reducing the risk of side effects like depression.

The benefits of l-arginine just keep stacking up. In addition to reducing heart disease, we are now learning more about how l-arginine helps the body release important hormones, increase lean muscle mass, speed wound recovery, and boost the immune system. Because l-arginine promotes healthy blood flow, it can also stimulate sexuality by decreasing impotence and female sexual dysfunction. There is also research to suggest that it can help Alzheimer's patients retard tumor growth, and help men with fertility problems.

You can get l-arginine from many types of foods, including dairy products, meat, fish, and chocolate. However, the average daily intake of l-arginine usually only meets the body's basic requirements for tissue repair and cell maintenance. L-arginine supplements provide much more of the amino acid available to your body for its many other purposes.

A typical supplement dose is about 2 grams a day, but in clinical trials of patients with congestive heart failure, as much as 15 grams a day has been successfully administered. I was able to reverse my atherosclerosis with only two 500mg doses a day. I now recommended more than that for my patients. The toxicity level for amino acids is 50 to 500 times the therapeutic dose range, so there is little danger of taking too much. However, high-dose l-arginine supplementation may result in watery diarrhea and sometimes stomach cramps and headaches. People with herpes and other viral infections should not take l-arginine supplements because it appears to promote the viral growth.

I believe that l-arginine is the single most important discovery in preventing heart disease that I have seen during the course of my medical career. Of course, there are many treatments for heart disease, but I haven't seen anything as effective. Pharmaceutical representatives for cholesterol-lowering statins get excited about a drug that shows a 30% success rate in lowering cholesterol. They tell me about their products and I say, "I think 99% is a pretty good success rate. What do you think?" There is a place for statins, but I don't think they are the most successful approach.

We cannot ignore the power of l-arginine any more. Heart disease is the number one killer in our country for both men and women. The main factors are arteriosclerosis, hardening of the arteries, and atherosclerosis, buildup on the arterial lining. L-arginine reverses both problems.

Nutraceuticals

Thanks to my success with l-arginine, I have made a gradual move to incorporating natural products into my treatment plans for patients. I have become a major advocate of nutraceuticals as part of total body care. Nutraceuticals are natural compounds, such as vitamins and minerals, omegas, and herbal extracts that can prevent, and in some cases even reverse, disease. You may sometimes hear nutraceuticals referred to as phytochemicals or functional foods. Nutraceuticals are substances that have health value beyond the traditional nutrients they contain.

Nutraceuticals are becoming more popular, as educated patients become increasingly proactive in pursuing wellness. Some people turn to nutraceuticals because they are justifiably frustrated with medicine that only treats disease. They want to prevent disease. Others are angered by the high cost of prescription drugs. Still, many others are drawn to nutraceuticals because they are hoping to reverse some aspects of the aging process, such as wrinkling of the skin or decrease in sex drive.

In order to understand nutraceuticals, you must understand the important role phytochemicals play in our bodies. We all know that we need food in order to supply our body with essential nutrients. Essential nutrients are the vitamins, minerals, fats, and proteins that we require in order to live. Unlike essential nutrients, we don't need phytochemicals to survive. However, phytochemicals are important because they protect us from diseases, including cancer and heart disease.

Phytochemicals come mostly from fruits and vegetables. You've been eating phytochemicals and nutraceuticals your whole life, but you might not have known it. Almost all plant foods contain nutraceuticals. Recently, products and supplements have been created and marketed that contain higher amounts of nutraceuticals than occur naturally in foods. Go into any supermarket and you are bound to see breakfast cereal touting "added isoflavones" or margarine that has cholesterol-lowering compounds. They can be valuable because they provide more important compounds than you could realistically expect to eat, even with a healthy diet. An acre of broccoli and a small dose of folic acid do the same thing; which would you rather have?

There are undoubtedly many nutraceuticals that we have not even discovered yet. I've already told you about l-arginine. Here is a breakdown of some other commonly known nutraceuticals that have been shown to lower your risk of a host of diseases:

- Isoflavones are found in soy foods and may reduce the risk of some cancers.

- Flavonoids are powerful antioxidants with hormonal properties. There are hundreds of compounds that can be considered flavonoids. A diet rich in flavonoids can protect the body against many types of cancer. While many vegetables and fruits are packed with flavonoids, some of the best sources of are tomatoes, kale, and onions.

- Lignans are found in flaxseed and rye. They have anti-estrogen properties that could reduce the risk of breast cancer.

- Indoles are found in cruciferous vegetables like broccoli. They may reduce the risk of estrogen-related cancers.

- Lycopene is a carotenoid that gives the red color to tomatoes, watermelon, and pink grapefruit. There is evidence that it can reduce the risk of multiple forms of cancer, including lung, bladder, prostate, cervix, and skin.

- Beta-carotene is a powerful antioxidant and cancer fighter. This is a phytochemical that most people know about. Sources include carrots, sweet potatoes, and leafy green vegetables.

- Lutein can reduce the risk of cancer and macular degeneration. Lutein may also help prevent atherosclerosis. The best sources include leafy green vegetables.

- Allyl sulfides help eliminate toxic compounds in the body. Best sources include onions, leeks, and scallions.

- Dithiolthiones and isothiocyanates can help the body detoxify cancer-causing compounds by increasing the activity of beneficial enzymes. Good sources include cruciferous vegetables, like broccoli, cauliflower, cabbage, and Brussels sprouts.

- Quercetin gives red apples and red onions their color. This anti-oxidant is a natural anti-inflammatory and anti-histamine. There is evidence that it can prevent some forms of cancer, including prostate.

There is another vitamin that we have heard about, but are only now starting to know its amazing ability to ward off disease. There is mounting evidence that vitamin D can help prevent many forms of cancer. About six years ago, doctors started to discover that patients given high doses of vitamin D experienced 80% less breast cancer and 90% less lung cancer! The problem is that the vast majority of us are not getting nearly enough vitamin D to experience its full benefits.

Vitamin D is found in foods, including fortified milk. Our body also makes vitamin D when we are exposed to sunlight. However, it is almost impossible to get a therapeutic dose from diet and sunlight alone. Plus, exposure to too much sunlight can increase the risk of skin cancer.

Years ago, the government decided how much vitamin D Americans should be getting and they began to add it to milk. That's why milk contains vitamin D. The problem is that their figures were way off. I believe that we should be getting about 3,000 IUs each day. Unfortunately, it is illegal to put that amount in something sold over-the-counter. You need a prescription to get the proper dosage of vitamin D. If you do take larger-than-recommended doses of vitamin D, it is very important to periodically monitor your blood levels to prevent toxicity. I am hoping this will change as the benefits of vitamin D become more widely understood and expected.

Overall, I am very pleased to see more people learn about various supplements, including manufactured nutraceuticals. However, I caution against taking any supplement before researching the product or talking with your physician. The amount of nutrients and amino acids you need is influenced by your gender, diet, and even where you live. What is right for someone else may be totally wrong for you.

Furthermore, don't fall into the trap of thinking that supplements are enough to maintain good health. Supplements cannot replace a balanced diet. Eat as many fruits and vegetables as you can. They are naturally rich in nutraceuticals. The supplement dose does not replace the broccoli.

CHAPTER 8

Total Body Wellness

Although total body wellness is common now, no one was talking about it when I received my diagnosis of atherosclerotic heart disease. Moreover, such a comprehensive approach, including the use of nutraceuticals, was completely different than anything I was taught at the University of California. At that time, all of the endocrinologists there said, "As you go out in the world and you become a practitioner, you must never stray outside the strict confines of what that disease of diabetes is. If you become known as someone who can help patients totally, you're will steal patients away from your referral source. So don't do it."

It didn't seem like good advice to give a physician. It may be the way things were done in another era, but I felt certain that I was not going to let anyone's health fail based on bad advice. After all, if I don't want to take that advice, why should my patients? From that point on, I treated the whole person, not just their disease. No system works independently in the body, so I believe it is often shortsighted to focus on only one system when it fails.

There's an old tradition in medicine. You don't ever ask a patient to do something that you wouldn't do yourself. I believe in that idea. However, I also believe you don't deny a patient a responsible course of treatment that you yourself would use. That's why I started telling my patients about l-arginine, even though many doctors frown on discussing natural medicine with their patients. They are too busy focusing on a patient's immediate or most pressing symptoms. I call this treating the "disease du jour."

I think it is important not to rule out any course of treatment that can have a positive impact on the patient. While I am a strong supporter of all of the wonderful advancements brought about by modern medicine, I also believe there is a place for natural or "alternative" treatments. The key is striking a balance. I've seen doctors completely dismiss any treatment that doesn't come out of a pharmacy bottle. I've also had patients who are resistant to explore anything they don't consider natural. Both approaches mystify me.

In many parts of the world, doctors are more willing to embrace alternative treatments. For instance, I've had the pleasure of discussing medical philosophies with doctors from Paris. They believe that if something works for a patient, it is important not to discount it, even if they do not fully understand why it is helpful. Therefore, it is not surprising to learn that many patients in France and other parts of Europe consult an herbalist; much the way Americans seek help from their pharmacists.

In the United States, these discoveries and theories are discarded under the category of miscellaneous scientific observation. American medical professionals believe in the double-blind approach to medical research.

Double-blind experiments are very stringent and are used to eliminate any subjective bias or expectation that the human subjects or the researchers may have. In a double-blind study, both the participants and the researchers are "blind," that is, neither knows which subjects are in the control group. Some volunteer subjects will receive the drug being researched; others will receive a similar looking placebo. The information regarding who is taking the drug is only released after the study is concluded and the results are known.

Double-blind experiments are an important part of scientific research. In fact, they are often best way to get the clearest answer to pressing questions. As a researcher, I have worked hard to keep my own intuitions and prejudice from clouding the outcome of my work and have found that double-blind experiments help facilitate objective results.

The problem with the double-blind approach when it comes to treating patients is that it forces medical professionals to devalue what intuition tells them might work. Previous experiences and intuition don't count for anything. Just because a conclusion about a treatment has been reached based on a scientific study doesn't mean that it is always accurate. Studies can have major flaws that are missed during the review process. Even if the study is accurate and unbiased, once the outcomes are published, the results can be misinterpreted.

The average person knows more about new medicines now than at any point in history, because people are bombarded by marketing, including television commercials, telling them to ask their doctors for certain prescription drugs. These marketing devices are influential. Most people do not know that the studies these drug companies mention in advertisements were carried out in a way that was heavily biased toward their product. I saw proof of this firsthand when I worked as a consultant for computer analysis companies that help develop pharmaceuticals.

The process is quite complicated, but basically boils down to computer modeling to achieve a desired outcome. Workers for these companies research everything they can find on a disease and put it into a computer program. Using this information, they determine which kind of study will best prove that a drug performs well. Even before they start the study, the outcome is decided. It's not illegal and it is technically not fraud, but it is not as scientific as it appears.

Our current scientific research process was incorporated into medicine because its rigor is important for the maintenance of good health. It is meant to safeguard people from treatments that could prove harmful. However, it has also led to a closed-minded and profit-centered approach to medicine. As a doctor, I have been faced with situations where I sat in a room with a patient and realized that there is no known scientific treatment that will help their problem. When confronted with this scenario, some doctors will just say, "I can't help you. There is no science that will work for you." I find this self-defeating to the patient and to the physician.

What I find even worse are health care professionals who will deny knowing about a certain treatment option.

For instance, a patient who asks about l-arginine might be told by her doctor, "I've never heard of it being used as a treatment. I don't know anything about it, so you should not take it." Later, we learn that the doctor is taking arginine, but just doesn't feel comfortable talking to his patients about alternative treatment options. This is a total disconnect. In fact, I have heard some doctors even go so far as to criticize other physicians for telling patients about remedies that are not considered mainstream. This is not an uncommon practice and it does not serve patient's interests.

I believe that while American scientific study is invaluable in many respects, personal experiences are also relevant, even if they run contrary to current medical beliefs. The best doctors are those who are not afraid to draw on the totality of their experiences. They acknowledge that there can be value in ideas that have yet to be proven. Given all the training doctors receive, they should be able to think anew about things, be open to alternative treatments, and constantly ask questions. They should not be afraid to give patients the information they need to make informed decisions about their own care.

The pendulum may swing too far the other way as well. Some patients distrust Western medicine. During the course of my career, I've had patients tell me, "I just don't want to have to take pills. I want to treat my diabetes with only a healthy diet and natural remedies." I say to them, "That may be a good start for you, but you should know that it may not be enough." One may not have to take pills forever. But, I suggest that they be open to medication until they become normal. Patients should not rule out anything that may help them to reverse their disease.

I am certain that we will gradually see a shift away from traditional Western medications and toward natural care. With this approach, everyone will have the power to help themselves by not only treating disease, but by preventing it and even reversing it. Your body has the power to rid itself of many diseases if you give it the tools it needs. The melding of natural and traditional medicine is the most exciting thing to happen in my professional experience.

Caring and Empathy

Dealing with my illness has made me more open to new treatment options. It has also helped me understand my patients better. I have more empathy for their struggles. When patients come into my office, I know that they are always at least a little bit worried. I investigate all of their symptoms thoroughly, even if those symptoms do not appear to be relevant to their specific complaints.

One of my patients recently died. I had been seeing her for about a year and a half and was saddened to hear of her passing. Her family called me to thank me for the care I had given her. They said she had gone to many different physicians over the years for various illnesses. Each doctor treated a specific problem, but none looked at her case from a total care perspective.

By looking at her entire medical history and discussing her lifestyle habits, I was able to eliminate the chronic, major suffering she experienced. Her thirty years of back pain disappeared. She was experiencing dementia, so I helped work out a solution where she wouldn't be alone all of the time. I wanted to make sure she was safe. This is not the usual role of an endocrinologist, but why should I let my "specialty" stop me from helping my patients in as many ways as possible?

My patient eventually died of lung cancer. In the end, there was no way to prevent her death. One of her family members told me, "We were so pleased with what you did. You treated all the things that made her feel bad and she returned to normal where possible. She had a better quality of life in the last year and a half than she had as long as we had known her."

Not only do I look at each case from a total care perspective, I also put my patients' symptoms in perspective for them. Usually, that means when I'm leaving the exam room I give a short speech. I reassure them by saying, "This is not serious. This will get better. We may not have the answers today but we're on our way," I am always honest and tell them that most therapies only work about 80% of the time. But if we fail, we'll try again with something different. I like to joke with my patients by saying, "I was wrong once, but I was very young. However, there's a good chance I'm going to be wrong one more time." The main thing is that I will keep trying until we have improved their quality of life as much as possible.

CHAPTER 9

The Value of Your Health

Today, information enters our realm in a fast-paced, abundant way. There is a concept that everybody can become their own best source of medical knowledge. It really makes it very important to understand there's a value to maintaining your health. Before you can take better care of yourself, start with an assessment of what you know about your health and what you consider most important to your well-being.

Start by asking yourself the value you place on the following:

Food

- What do you eat?
- How do you eat?
- When do you eat?
- Why do you eat?

Exercise

- How much exercise do you get?
- What types of exercise do you perform?
- What types of exercise works best for your body type?

- When do you exercise?

Stress Management

- How does your body react to stress?
- How do you recognize stress?
- How do you calm yourself?
- How you know the difference between coping with life and effectively managing you life? This is an important distinction. You can cope in a variety of unhealthy ways, such as overeating, but to truly manage your life you must handle stress in a way that benefits your body as well as your mind.

Quality of Life

- How would you rate the quality of your life?
- What factors affect your quality of life?
- How much are you willing to change to improve your quality of life?

Self-Care

A few years ago, I went to a large medical meeting attended by several hundred executives of the largest companies in the United States. The subject turned to educating employees on health issues. The human resources director from a well known Fortune 500 company said, "There are about 30% of our employees that will not know what to do with the health education we give them. We need to shepherd them in this endeavor." Everyone in the place went silent. Finally a voice from the back of the room shouted, "Do you mean you've hired a staff for your company that you cannot educate?" It brought the house down.

While this story may be humorous, it is a prime example of the tendency of those in charge to underestimate the people they serve. This happens in medicine as much as any other discipline. When I first started working in the field of diabetes, it was widely assumed that patients would not be able to make the significant lifestyle changes necessary to improve their health. Many doctors did not give their patients credit for what they could do; so they didn't even bother to give them the knowledge they needed to best take care of themselves.

I become angry when I hear health care professionals make comments like, "Our patients will never be able to do this…" I say, "Of course they can. Give people the tools they need to improve their health. Some people may not change their habits, but many more will rise to the occasion."

I am a firm believer in patient responsibility and self-care. Patients want and deserve the opportunity to do better. Sadly, many physicians do not stress self-care enough and many patients never take control of their health. I try to explain to all of my patients that in order to be healthy, they must participate in their own health care.

Self-care has played an important role in my own family's lifestyle. Like all parents, my wife, Marlene, and I have passed on genetic traits to our children. Some of those traits make them more susceptible to particular diseases. For instance Marlene has increased levels of homocysteine, an amino acid present in everyone. However, if you have a genetic trait that causes an increased level of homocysteine, you run a much higher risk of having a heart attack in your 50s or 60s.

I first learned about homocysteine when I was going through medical school. Like a lot of students, I brought my newfound knowledge home and tried to use it to benefit those I cared about. Because of high incidence of heart disease in her family, I tested Marlene and found that she had homocysteine levels that were higher than normal. I immediately suggested she take high levels of folic acid to prevent her condition from causing health problems in the future. She agreed and has been taking a daily dose of folic acid ever since.

Knowing that the problem is largely genetic, I gave

the same advice to Marlene's father and brother. They asked their doctors if they should begin taking folic acid, but the doctors simply scoffed at the idea. Because they trusted their physicians, both my brother-in-law and father-in-law did not attempt to monitor or control their homocysteine levels. They also never gave folic acid a second thought. Sadly, my father-in-law later died of a heart attack. Marlene's brother suffered a heart attack that he was fortunate enough to survive. Meanwhile, my wife has no signs of heart disease, thanks in large part to the folic acid supplements she takes.

Despite the success of folic acid, many cardiologists are not convinced that it is a worthwhile treatment. In fact, many believe there is not sufficient proof that homocysteine even causes heart problems. Homocysteine simply doesn't fit into the neat box required by current scientific study. However, I believe that truth can be often be found by searching for solutions outside of that box. Just because the link between homocysteine levels and heart attacks cannot be fully explained does not mean that the link does not exist. It may ultimately be a link to something like the metabolic syndrome that causes the heart disease and only secondarily raises the homocysteine. Those with elevated homocysteine levels do not have an additional 20 years to unwrap this mystery, so they should be given the information that we do know so that they can make an informed decision about what they want to do.

My family has refused to allow this type of narrow thinking dictate how we protect ourselves from disease. I think everyone should be checked for a variety of genetic mutations, including homocysteine. One in eleven people have high levels of homocysteine, yet the vast majority of these people have never even heard of it. I routinely put all of my patients over age 18 through a battery of tests to discover what risks they may have. I checked my own children for increased levels of homocysteine once they became adults. My daughter is fine, but my son has the same problem as his mother. He started taking folic acid in his early 20s while still in college.

My son is now married to a lovely woman. When she first met us, she asked me to tell her about our family. I suppose she wanted a description of where we had lived and what the kids had been like while growing up. I told her that stuff, but I also launched into a discussion about our various medical conditions. She laughingly responded, "Good God! What am I getting into?" I said, "Yes, we are a genetic cesspool, but at least we know what is in that cesspool and we are dealing with it."

The truth is everyone carries traits from their genetic cesspools that make them more susceptible to disease. The difference is that my family has actively sought the knowledge necessary to protect our health. Part of self-care is refusing to stick your head in the sand. You can't ward off conditions you don't know about.

Knowing your family's medical history does not mean that you have a crystal ball that allows you to see your future. Having a family history of a disease does not mean that you are automatically going to get it to. We are not victims of our genes. We control our own lives. It is important to know that there is a big difference between knowing what you might be facing and resigning yourself to disease. Use your knowledge about your family history as a tool to empower yourself into practicing improved self-care. Your lifestyle plays a major role in determining what diseases and medical conditions you will experience. You may not be able to change your genetics, but you can change the way you eat, exercise, and manage stress.

Challenges and Self-Care Solutions

At this time in medical history, health care is largely set up for the treatment of disease. I believe we need to work on the flip side of standard health care. Thus being a self-care advocate may mean bucking the system. It is far more important to know what the risks of developing diseases are, and then prevent them in the first place. Patients are not interested in getting a disease and then being treated; they are interested in doing what they can to never get the disease.

Why don't more doctors embrace the idea of self-care? I have worked with hundreds of health care professionals and almost all of them are committed to serving their patients in the best way possible. In other words, their hearts are in the right place. If asked, most doctors would agree that they would rather deal with a knowledgeable patient than a passive one not engaged in his or her own health. However, a patient who is savvy about self-care can threaten a doctor by using their newfound knowledge to go against the doctor's advice. Educated patients are also more likely to ask more demanding questions and take it upon themselves to look beyond traditional medicine and try alternative treatments.

I believe that self-care is a basic, elementary idea. Yet, most Americans have no experience with this. In the health class you took as a kid (if you even had a regular health class), you were probably taught a narrow lesson plan involving the names of the bones in the body and how the organs work. This is educational, but not nearly as practical as teaching young people about the common illnesses and diseases that affect them and their families.

Schools should teach students how their diet and exercise habits will affect their bodies throughout their lives. Memorizing the USDA Food Pyramid is not enough. Students need to understand the ramifications of the average American diet on a body. Classes should also address consumer issues, so students know that they cannot be passive about their health. All young people are smart enough to know they should engage in activities that support good health. They deserve to know that when they are not feeling well, it is up to them to work toward reversing their illness.

Currently, I'm taking the idea of self-care to the next step by introducing medical centers where patients can walk in and have basic health screenings. Hopefully, they won't even need to make appointment to see a physician. This type of self-care center could be especially helpful for diabetics who must rely on regular testing for complications and monitoring of their blood glucose levels. I see this as a way to provide people with another tool to help them take control of their own health care.

Self-Care in Families

Marlene and I have always stressed the importance of self-care to our children. I've already discussed how I have tested them for potential problems. However, the best self-care does not come only from a medical test. It comes from how we live our daily lives.

From an early age, we taught our children the importance of eating well and having daily exercise. Marlene and I believe in teaching by example. When we ate well, our children ate well. By seeing us engage in exercise, they came to accept physical activity as an essential part of life. We also spent time talking about how to keep our metabolisms at their absolute peak. Our children grew up with an understanding that their bodies should be respected and cared for.

Marlene and I have learned to be flexible in both how we care for ourselves and our family. We value the wisdom we glean from our life experiences and from the input of others. Still, we are constantly re-evaluating what we have learned and are always ready to discard an idea or activity if it does not work for us. We tried to teach our children to be independent thinkers. Sometimes you have to be willing to run away from something that seems pretty good in search of something else that may be better. This applies not only to how we care for our physical health, but also how we take care of our emotional well-being.

Emotional Self-Care

All illnesses take a psychological as well as a physical toll on the patient. This is especially true for diabetics. Many diabetics get impatient with the constant monitoring and grow frustrated with trying to cope with the lifestyle changes required to maintain good health. New patients can find the process overwhelming. Others get off to a good start and then find it hard to stick to the daily regimen. Even though they know their health is on the line, they find it difficult to muster the motivation to keep going. I've also seen patients who are doing great with their self-care become depressed when their glucose levels fluctuate, despite following all of the "rules." It is hard to stay the course when you are not rewarded with success.

I explain to my patients that diabetes is not just about physical health. It is also about honoring your emotions. It is normal to feel angry, burnt out, and sad. The key is to acknowledge how you feel, but still manage to keep yourself focused on the larger picture.

I talk with patients about what keeps them from a positive attitude. Is it high blood glucose test results? Is it not being able to overindulge on food during the holidays? Is it the realization that this is a lifelong battle? We then brainstorm about ways to tackle their problems. We focus on the easier issues first so he or she can experience the satisfaction of overcoming an obstacle. Sometimes fixing a little problem can make the bigger issues seem more manageable.

Stress and diabetes can create a dangerous circle. Managing diabetes can be stressful, and that stress can worsen the condition. When you are stressed, your body starts producing stress hormones like cortisol and epinephrine. Those hormones raise your blood sugar in an effort to provide the body with the energy necessary to "fight or flight." However, a rapid increase in blood sugar can adversely affect diabetics. If stress becomes a chronic problem, it aggravates the many complications associated with diabetes, including blindness, nerve damage, and kidney problems.

It is crucial that patients recognize when they are under stress. It is easy to notice stress during major life events, such as moving or experiencing a divorce. It is harder to pick up smaller, constant stresses, like work problems or taking care of a household. Stress can become so much a part of our everyday existence that we don't even notice that our bodies are under attack. I tell my patients to be more in tune with their feelings. It helps to make a note of their emotions each time they check their blood sugar. It surprises a lot of people to see just how much daily stressors can affect their glucose levels.

Once we've narrowed down what is causing stress, we can work on ways to relax. Great ways to combat frayed nerves include any form of physical activity, relaxing hobbies, and meditation. When you feel stress coming on, one of the best things to do is to simply step away from the situation and engage in some breathing exercises. That moment of acknowledging the stress and relieving it can have an immediate calming effect.

Support Systems

Self-care is often considered something that involves only the individual. However, self-care can involve support networks, including friends, families, church organizations, and community groups. I routinely encourage patients to ask for support from the people they are close to. Requesting help in a difficult situation is a sign of emotional intelligence, not a sign of weakness. For instance, I might say, "Look, you have demonstrated a lack of self-control when it comes to sweets. Don't feel bad about it or deny it. Just work on it. Tell those folks at the office not to put the pan of brownies near your desk. They will honor your wishes."

There are many ways to seek out people who share your interest in healthy living. One way is to find a workout partner. You are much less likely to skip an exercise session if you know a friend is waiting for you. Taking low-fat cooking classes can also be a fun way of making friends who will encourage your new enthusiasm for better nutrition.

Sometimes people will try to help you in ways that feel intrusive or inappropriate. Perhaps your brother generously gives you his old treadmill, but then makes comments that you don't look like you are using it enough. Your spouse might go along with your request not to buy junk food, but then comment on everything you put into your mouth. What is meant to be supportive can sometimes make the diabetic feel embarrassed or criticized.

Instead of being angry and resentful, thank the person for caring enough to offer you advice. Even if you are offended, you do not want to alienate those you love. Explain exactly how they can support you in a better way. Be direct and specific. For example, you might say, "Honey, when you comment on my weight, it makes me feel discouraged. I know you want to help me, and I really value your encouragement and support. Would you be willing to watch the kids for a half hour every morning so I can exercise before work?" If your spouse regularly cooks foods that are fattening or unhealthy, you may have to request very directly that they change their cooking style or at least understand when you no longer eat it.

I encourage my patients to educate their loved ones about their disease. Family members need to understand that treatment plans take time to work and fluctuations in blood glucose levels are common. It is counterproductive for family members to criticize the patient for not controlling glucose levels. Even patients who are very strict with their diet and exercise programs experience ups and downs. Criticizing leads to feelings of isolation, anger, and resentment. Family members help the most when they focus on acceptable ways to encourage and support the patient.

Support groups can be helpful to people dealing with illness and self-care. My diabetic patients in support groups say that they learn from hearing about the experiences of others and are also grateful to be able to share their own struggles with people who understand what they are going through. Doctors and other health care staff do not usually attend support groups. This allows members of the group to speak freely about their treatment experiences. Patients who reach out to others are more likely to embrace the lifestyle changes necessary to treat their disease.

The Internet provides online support groups for diabetes and most other illnesses. Patients can discuss common problems and solutions and get emotional support from their "virtual" friends. The educational process on the web groups is that once a discussion is initiated on a message board, even those not involved in the "conversation" can read the text and gain from it. In this way, thousands of people have access to valuable information without having to participate, which is important to people who don't wish to ask directly for help or want to stay anonymous. I am such a strong advocate of Internet support that I have included online discussion boards as part of my Diabetes One-on-One Program at http://www.diabetesoneonone.com/community/.

For some patients, the emotional consequences of diabetes are far more serious than normal, everyday frustrations. Diabetics are more likely than the average person to suffer from depression. People with diabetes can feel helpless, which is one of the major emotions that contribute to depression. It is normal for patients to go through periods of sadness. However, if the sadness lasts for more than a few weeks, it is important to seek professional help.

It is important that diabetics pay attention to mental health. This is an essential part of self-care. Doctors may fail to recognize depression in their patients. Sometimes patients are too embarrassed to truthfully answer questions. Either way, too many diabetics are not getting the help they need for their clinical depression.

It is imperative to see a mental health professional when you experience these symptoms lasting for more than two weeks:

- Feelings of sadness that last for most of the day

- Less interest in things you used to enjoy

- Feeling no pleasure from things that normally would make you happy

- Irregular sleep patterns

- Rapid weight gain or loss (this is especially dangerous for diabetics)

- Thoughts of death or suicide

- Inability to focus on daily tasks or to concentrate on work

There are many options available to treat depression. If you are experiencing the symptoms listed above, do not wait to get help.

Communicating With Your Doctor

Part of self-care is knowing when to seek professional treatment and how to ask the right questions once you get there. As a patient, you can't always depend on your health care providers to give you all of the information you require. You have to be an advocate for yourself. Remember, you will not be able to make the right choices about your health if you don't know what the options are.

Whether you are dealing with a physical or emotional problem, don't expect your doctor to tell you everything you might want to know. And don't rely on your doctors to ask you everything they need to know! If you suspect your physician does not fully understand your situation, you need to communicate with them effectively until they know exactly what you are experiencing. Here is a list of ways to make the most out of your time with your health care provider.

Tell your doctor about:

- Any symptoms you are experiencing, even if they don't seem connected to the illness you are seeking treatment for

- Health conditions that run in your family, including diabetes, heart disease, cancer, and high blood pressure

- Any past medical problems you have had

- Any medications you currently take

Things to ask your doctor about (write down the answers):

- Why you have your illness?

- What course of treatment to follow?

- What happens if you forget to follow the treatment or take your medication?

- How long your treatment will last?

- How you should handle your symptoms?

- Under what conditions should you seek emergency treatment?

- When you should return for your next appointment?

- Where you can get more information about your condition?

- Where can you get a second opinion?

Navigating the Constantly Changing Health Care System

It is estimated that there are 16 million patients with diabetes and only 5,000 endocrinologists. Of these, only 3,500 endocrinologists are in full time practice and diabetes care only encompasses about 50% of their patient population. Thus, primary care physicians care for the vast majority of people with diabetes. For many patients, the selection of primary care physicians is severely restricted by insurance plans. While this does not necessarily have to be a problem, it is important that the patient understand the drawbacks of such a system.

The main problem is that primary care physicians are required to be jack-of-all-trades. They must know about an almost-unending list of diseases and conditions. While they may be perfectly qualified to help a diabetic with basic concerns, they may not always be aware of the newest research and treatment options. I believe patients benefit from a team of health care professionals working for them, including a primary care physician, endocrinologist, dietitian, education support staff, physiologist (to help with exercise), and a psychologist, if necessary.

A number of studies to date have demonstrated improved outcomes when patients receive care from specialists. A recent survey, published by Washington Hospital Center, found that most primary care physicians don't provide appropriate annual examinations to determine whether their patients' diabetes is well-managed. In many cases, the patients are left on their own to make difficult decisions about a complex medical problem. As a result, these patients have a higher chance of developing complications that can be severe and life threatening.

Patients must be very knowledgeable and persistent to get the best care possible. Here are some things to keep in mind if your insurance company limits you to a primary care physician:

Carefully choose your primary care physician. You want a doctor who understands your illness, and who has a working relationship with specialists that you can go to if necessary.

Take the time to understand your insurance policy. Know what you have a right to ask for and what coverage may be denied.

Don't be afraid to advocate for services. If you think you should be receiving a course of treatment that insurance won't cover, pursue your case. Let them know that paying for preventative medicine now will keep you from developing costly medical problems in the future.

Understand that you may have to pay for some services out of pocket, including visits to another doctor if you want a second opinion.

If you are unhappy with your physician but feel you have limited options because of your insurance, contact your local diabetes association for help. They may be able to help you locate a different doctor. Also, let your employer or insurer know that you are dissatisfied with the available resources. Employers can pick new insurance carriers based on feedback.

Self-care is especially important for people with diabetes because they must perform regular testing and observe their bodies to manage the disease. A comprehensive self-care approach to wellness means that diabetics will rely less on doctors and emergency services. Self-care makes for healthier patients, and it is also cost-effective.

Remember that it is your responsibility to be healthy. It is your choice to live longer. Don't deprive yourself of knowledge. You deserve to enjoy the many benefits of having a healthy body.

But the present system won't pay for most of this despite what the brochure said when you signed up. The system is not working and it is not delivering a value for the exorbitant cost.

At the heart of the matter is the deep belief that someone else should pay for your health care. It has grown to be a major problem for the nation. Even though it is a tax deduction for the employer, companies are struggling with the increasing costs. The President's Advisory Panel on Federal Tax Reform has named health care by far the most expensive deduction in the tax code. However, the extraordinary costs have not produced an especially healthy population in the United States. Newt Gingrich has said we have turned the health care system into a rental car and nobody bothers to wash a rental car.

I gave a speech in Singapore on Labor Day weekend 2005. A gentleman pulled up a chair next to me before my speech and said, "We have a tradition in Asia of health with natural products. We will keep that tradition because it emphasizes wellness. The United States has a system of sickness, of treating disease rather than pursuing health. You have come to tell us how to take our tradition into the next century. We look forward to what you say."

The insurance companies can take 11% of the claims they handle. This is money they then use to refine the software that "denies" most of the claims that are submitted from diabetics. They have already lost the first round in court on this issue, but I don't see that causing a fundamental change. As Newt Gingrich said "so we are not going to cover your preventive care but we will pay for your dialysis when you are 45." What kind of a health care system is that?" It's not cost effective and it is certainly not good for the health of all Americans.

We need a system that identifies those at risk and begins reversal therapy. I do this every day. It is not the standard in the realm of endocrinology and metabolism, and certainly not in the subset of diabetes.

CHAPTER 10

Reaching Out Through Telemedicine

The great American inventor, Thomas Edison, once predicted, "The doctor of the future will give no medicine, but will interest patients in the maintenance of the human frame, in diet and in the prevention of disease." This is my goal, and I hope Edison's prediction will come true. Unfortunately, it hasn't happened yet. Although most of Western medicine is still focused primarily on disease treatment, there are shifts towards disease prevention through total body and self-care. One of the most exciting trends is the use of the Internet to reach underserved populations and provide access to information about health and wellness.

About 15 years ago, I got my first glimpse of how the Internet could change the way we treat patients. I had been using the online archives of the Library of Congress as part of my medical research. At that time, the system wasn't very streamlined and it took a lot of time to wade through information. One day, I received a phone call from one of my medical practice partners. He had a patient who had a bad thyroid problem and he said, "Unless you can think of some something else, we will have to evaluate him for a heart transplant at Stanford on Monday."

I immediately thought of the online research I had just been reading. I went back online and found two articles about cutting-edge thyroid treatments that a few people were performing. We instituted those treatments and instead of being evaluated for a transplant on Monday, the patient went home on Wednesday.

The Internet is part of our everyday lives, yet its applications in health care still remain largely untapped. Although there are thousands of health-related websites, we can do much more with this incredible tool. I have spent the last ten years working to use the Internet as a way to reach people who suffer from chronic illnesses such as diabetes.

It is less expensive to connect with people via the Internet than to establish practices and build buildings. If people have instant access to the education they need to take care of themselves, we can reverse their illnesses and, at the same time, lower the skyrocketing costs associated with traditional health care.

Exciting technology is already available, and more is on the way. There are monitoring devices that allow diabetic patients to test their blood glucose levels and send the results to their health care provider over the Internet. There are also special shirts that can transmit cardiovascular information, including heart and respiratory rate, to our computers. Although these devices are not in widespread use now, their development is part of an important trend.

Sadly, I see disconnect between patients' willingness to use the Internet and doctors' willingness to communicate with them the same way. Most people today use the Internet to research health information. They would find it convenient to email their physicians when necessary. However, many doctors remain resistant to Internet health care. Some have told me too much of the information on the web is inaccurate and patients are misinformed. Doctors also feel that they have hectic schedules that do not allow them time to respond to emails or take part in Internet-based treatment plans. I understand their concerns, but I think they are shortsighted. After all, the same thing happened with the telephone.

At the turn of the last century, the telephone was an exciting new invention. Many industries embraced the technology, but doctors, as a whole, did not. Many assumed that time with patients would be reduced if they had to answer phone calls during the day. Others were convinced that patients would never be able to learn to use the telephone, so it wasn't valuable. You know the rest of the story. We all ended up with telephones and now no one thinks twice about calling their doctor's office to make an appointment or ask a question. I think in time we won't remember when we didn't communicate with our doctors via the Internet.

Telemedicine in Action

I started my company, Endocrine Therapeutics, because I see the potential and power of the Internet. The company provides professional medical services to clinics and hospitals, with a specific interest in online interaction as a way serve the diabetes community. In order to directly reach patients with diabetes, I also started the Diabetes One-on-One Program in 1994. The program offers treatment, support, and education geared toward helping people gain control over their disease. Keeping people informed about new concepts and treatments can empower patients to take action, resulting in the reversal of many metabolic complications.

When I started the company, I was very excited, but unsure of exactly how the program would work. It was somewhat uncharted territory. Once we resolved the technical aspects, the rest fell together nicely according to my vision.

Today, Endocrine Metabolic Medical Center's role is to deliver the care to patients as any doctor's office would do. Endocrine Therapeutics, Inc. is a company that develops the new technologies, gets new contracts for EMMC to deliver medical care, and is the publisher of all the protocols, educational material and books such as this one. EMMC employs the diabetes nurse educators (RNs) who take charge of managing patients' diabetes care with regular contact. An RN assesses a patient's health history by questions via email, phone, or fax. A medical record is assembled electronically that allows transmission of all the information to whomever, wherever, and whenever the patient deems appropriate. Video conferencing with the patient and RN is available, and is the favored communication mode.

Through this program, we provide complete diabetes care. We take care of medication changes, new prescriptions, dosage changes, and lab orders electronically. We review glucose updates and evaluate other symptom updates on-line. Like any office consultation, all lab and treatment changes are forwarded to the patient's physician. The participant must still visit a doctor periodically for blood pressure checks and physical exams. Otherwise, we do all that is necessary to integrate their diabetes with the rest of their lives. We provide access to online discussion groups, design appropriate exercise programs and dietary guidelines, and inform patients about new technologies that might benefit them. We even send weekly diabetes e-newsletters to patients and their doctors.

Promotora Program

Although my Internet outreach programs have been successful, participants have tended to be middle-class diabetic patients who already have a basic understanding of their disease and how to take care of themselves. It has troubled me that the underserved people who need a telemedicine program the most have had no way to access this type of service. Therefore, I have started the Promotora Telemedicine Project to reach out to the medically underserved community. The program was established in conjunction with the Pacific Medical Research Foundation.

Over the years, I have become increasingly concerned with the issue of diabetes in the Mexican-American population. Research suggests that the prevalence of diabetes in this group of Americans is reaching epidemic proportions. According to the CDC, Hispanic adults, including Mexican-Americans, are being diagnosed with diabetes at twice the rate of white Americans. About 25% of all Mexican-Americans between the ages of 45 and 74 have Type 2 diabetes. Younger Mexican-Americans, including children, are developing the disease. Once they develop the disease, Mexican-Americans tend to have more serious complications. For instance, they are about five times more likely to develop kidney failure, and they also have disproportionately high rates of diabetes-caused blindness.

There are specific factors behind this trend. A Baylor College of Medicine study concluded that Mexican-Americans might be genetically more susceptible to diabetes than other ethnic groups. According to the study, even healthy Mexican-Americans with no previously known risk factors for diabetes are more likely to have a metabolic abnormality that can lead to insulin resistance. Insulin resistance is the leading cause of more than 90% of diabetes in Mexican-Americans. Combine a genetic propensity to develop the disease with the high fat diet typical in America, and chances of developing diabetes increases dramatically.

The problem is not entirely based in genetics. There are social issues to be addressed to combat diabetes among Mexican-Americans. Lack of health insurance is a major barrier. In Santa Clara County, California, nearly 25% of Mexican-Americans do not have any form of medical coverage. This presents problems because diabetes requires more complicated treatment plans than other chronic diseases. My research has shown that diabetic patients in Santa Clara County who don't have insurance typically have to wait more than six months to get an intake appointment at the county's medical center. After that first appointment, they are not able to see a doctor as often as they should for follow-up treatment and monitoring.

Language barriers, lack of education, and cultural differences only exacerbate the problem. Even the best treatments are useless if the patient does not understand how to apply them. I wondered how we could use available technology in a culturally-sensitive way in order to break down some of these roadblocks.

My earlier work had proven that the Internet could not only improve quality of care for patients, but also lower health care costs. As president of the Endocrine Metabolic Center in Redwood City, California, I wanted to take what I had learned and use my resources to further serve members of a largely ignored community. That's how the Promotora Telemedicine Project was born.

We've now connected with free medical clinics in the region. They see patients who are working poor, meaning their jobs do not provide health insurance and they don't qualify for government programs. Some of these patients are recent immigrants and speak no English. Our first location was the RotaCare Bay Area Clinic in San Jose. At RotaCare clinics, all of the doctors and most of the staff are volunteers. They do an amazing job and should be commended for the long hours they spend. However, as volunteers, they have limited time for appointments and most do not specialize in diabetes.

We have recruited "promotora." They are bilingual, community-based facilitators. Most of them have no previous medical training, so we educate them on diabetes prevention and treatment. The promotora basically says to the patient, "I'm not a doctor but I am here to help speak English or Spanish to the doctor or nurse, I will tell them what you would like and get your questions answered."

During a telemedicine session, the promotora sits

beside the patient during the appointment, which is done through a two-way videoconferencing system. The promotora collects basic information about the patient's weight and vital signs. At the appointed time, the doctor or Certified Diabetes Educator connects to the system, allowing the patient and professional to see each other and speak through the promotora. The physician or educator electronically reviews the patient's information and provides a treatment plan, including diet, exercise, glucose monitoring information, and instructions for taking medicine if necessary. The session ends with the patient receiving medication, instructions written in Spanish, and an appointment card for the next visit.

Our diabetes team does not have to spend time traveling to each location, so we can reach many more people this way. Doctors who do not have the time or resources for extended office hours can administer to patients in workplaces, schools, and clinics without ever leaving their own home or office. The program has worked well and is starting to become nationally recognized. In February 2004, the American Medical Association gave me the Award for Excellence in Eliminating Health Disparities based on my development of the promotora program.

Telemedicine has its limitations. Some types of treatment require direct observation and touching. But volunteer doctors and nurses staff the RotaCare Clinic in San Jose every Wednesday evening. We schedule the telemedicine appointments on Wednesday afternoons. That way, if it is determined that the patient needs to have a "hands-on" appointment, they can stay for the clinic's evening hours and meet with a physician.

In the future, this same model may be useful for AIDS treatment in Africa. It is now being adapted by several Asian countries for rural care. The United State Congress has just adopted legislation to have a Telemedicine Center in the central United States. Health care workers can go anywhere with a solar powered personal computer, allowing them to give expert care to people, even in some of the world's most remote locations. The concept is the same whether the mobile telemedicine station is located in Ethiopia or downtown San Jose.

Telemedicine fills an important void in our society. It is effective where health care access is limited. This happens in rural and urban areas because of the large populations who do not have insurance or enough money to pay for traditional doctor visits. Telemedicine addresses these issues by providing high-quality care in an innovative and cost-effective way.

Conclusion

Often, I am called a "visionary." It may not be meant as a compliment. As I wrote this book, I considered the meaning of it. A visionary looks ahead. In that respect, I think all of us have the ability to be visionaries.

Curiosity has fueled my entire career. I am curious about health care and our common experiences as humans on this planet. I have a sense of wonder at all there is to learn and all that will remain forever a mystery. This curiosity has served me well, both professionally and personally. Without curiosity about atherosclerosis, I would not have started taking l-arginine, which improved my health and eventually the health of hundreds of my patients.

Today, when I see a patient, I am representing not only everything I have done in my life, but everything I want to become. I sometimes ask patients to look ahead 20 years. Many of them laugh and say, "Gee, in 20 years, I'll be dead!" I never think about my life or patients' lives in those terms. We are living longer now than we ever have in the history of mankind, so why not plan to be in the best psychological and physical shape possible and enjoy all those years? I encourage my patients to enjoy the remaining years and to never stop looking to the possibilities for the future. That's what makes a person a visionary.

My life experiences have also been shaped by skepticism. I always keep a little doubt in my mind about what I have learned. I never assume that work done before mine was done correctly. Diabetics used to be advised to eat a high-fat diet. Then, they were told to avoid all sugar. Now we know that fatty diets should be avoided, and it is not the simply the sugar that kills diabetics. That does not mean that everything we learn about medicine will ultimately be proven useless. But it likely means that someone may discover that our work was based on faulty assumptions.

True visionaries are leaders, and leaders lead. There are many times when we must follow certain rules. But I remain wary of the tyranny of conformity. This is a pivotal concept that prompts me to think unlike many other doctors. Traditional medicine would have treated my heart disease with prescription medication. Had I done that, I would still be treating that disease. Instead I reversed my disease.

You may be a leader too. As leaders, we have a moral duty to be a little revolutionary. When I started my work in diabetes, no one predicted we would come so far in understanding the disease. We haven't eradicated diabetes yet, but it is possible. No matter what your goal is, aim high. If you fail, as I have failed at various points in my life, fail with something really important and ahead of its time. Be a pioneer. Get out in front. The middle ground is an exposed, dangerous, and ungrateful position.

Being a visionary can be a lonely quest. Whether you are trying to cure a disease or organize a fundraiser for your church, true pioneers approach their projects with innovation that is often confounding to others. Be prepared. Your creativity might prompt your friends, family, and colleagues to view you strangely. Do not be deterred. As you take charge of your self-care program or start new projects, you cannot be assured that the action is right. But a smaller mind would never have started the project. I pioneered the idea of Internet-based telemedicine before many people were even comfortable with the idea of using a personal computer. Some physicians are still afraid of the idea. Yet, I know reaching the underserved population in our country is going to take a combination of innovation and new technology, especially as diabetes affects more and more people, health care costs are inaccessible, and more people have no medical insurance.

Believe in your vision. Set an example, and never ask people to do something you would not do yourself. Pursue social change by living it. Listen to both your followers and detractors. Don't be arrogant; they may be right. Don't let criticism deter you, and remember whom you serve. I serve those with diabetes. They have a stake in me staying the course for good health care. I carry with me the burden of what diabetics need. This altruistic sense has shaped my very existence and filled my life with passion and satisfaction.

When you are dealing with a health issue, keep working toward a solution. Do not back away from any challenge that is worth overcoming. A former Cranbrook School master, Mr. Robert Hoffman, taught me this expression: *Non illegitimus carborundum.* He translated it to mean, "Don't let the bastards wear you down." It is easy to conform or give into illness, but remember, if you do, you lose something beyond your health. It is your time.

INDEX

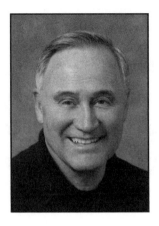

Dr. John Joseph Prendergast, a renaissance man, is an accomplished physician and humanist. As a young man, he overcame a learning disability, and gained compassion. As an adult, he sought relief for his physical health problems, and has empowered countless patients in the art of self-care for more than thirty years. The physician's tireless, ground-breaking work on diabetes has won him numerous awards. For the first time, Dr. Joe explains how he achieved success and explains how the lessons he has learned can apply to all of our lives.